HEALTHY NATURAL DIET
THE HND METHOD

DR. MARIANO MARINO

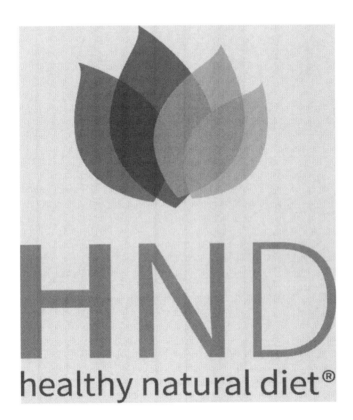

HND
healthy natural diet®

Contents

PREFACE

Healthy Natural Diet (HND) is an innovative and revolutionary dietary method in the field of nutrition. This method brings excellent physical health and wellness benefits.

HND is a totally natural vegetable based diet that is compatible with the anatomy and physiology of the human body: it excludes all processed foods such as, simple sugars, hydrogenated fats, animal proteins, preservatives, dyes, thickeners, stabilizers and various additives, and only includes nutrient dense foods that feed, satiate and bring energy and vitality to the body.

The most common diets are based mainly on calorie reduction and/or on the increase of protein, while neglecting the nutritional quality, or lack thereof, within those calories.

The principle of considering exclusively calories, carbohydrates, proteins or fats is already passed: without checking the quality of foods, not only are there no benefits in the long term, but the development of physical problems could occur, mainly caused by non-natural foods that are pro-inflammatory.

One's diet should not be intended as an effort or a sacrifice, but as a pleasure resulting from the awareness of making the right lifestyle choices.

By adopting some simple rules, dictated by the observance of circadian cycles of the body and by the quality of food choice, it becomes possible to change one's diet and finally reach the ideal weight, which will then not be a goal, but a consequence of healthy eating.

The HND method not only considers a healthy and natural nutrition, but it represents a true lifestyle, that includes regular physical activity balanced with one's e personal characteristics and goals, beyond the training level.

The HND method has different types of activities, aimed at training all muscles groups as well as the metabolic system.

The HND method consists of the ideal functional training, floor routines and equipment workouts to improve and/or regain the natural mobility, starting from competitive sports and useful daily practices, with the purpose of avoiding ailments and problems, frequently affecting a sedentary lifestyle.

Having a toned and flexible body enhances our overall appearance, our energy and well-being.

The HND method is suitable for everyone: for people with pathologies looking for healing, as well as athletes, and professionals that want to improve and optimize their performance.

Eating healthy and getting fit are the only true goals that you can achieve through our Healthy Natural Diet program.

INTRODUCTION

Today, overweight and obesity-related issues have become more and more alarming and out of control.

In fact, they represent the main cause for metabolic imbalances eventually leading to chronic diseases.

Moreover, many pathologies are found to be related in some way to nutrition: specifically diabetes, dyslipidaemias, cardiovascular diseases, as well as hepatic, renal and metabolic diseases in general are connected to the consumption of "junk" food, loaded with added sugars, low quality fats, animal proteins, preservatives, dyes, thickeners, stabilizers and various additives. [1,2,3,4]

Clinically speaking, the nutrients that create and enhance flavors are sugars and fats. Numerous studies have highlighted strong addiction to sugar in humans, sometime higher than some types of drugs. [5,6,7]

What follows is a continued consumption of "sugary" foods: if we eat food with "added" sugars, we become dependent on them. This addiction is difficult to interrupt. In fact, each time we eat food with added sugar we do nothing but strengthen it.

It is interesting to note how the industrialized food system (places that serve food, sell food and especially the mass media), promotes these kinds of food as good, tasteful and useful, advertising their consumption and neglecting to highlight the dark side that hides there.

If a product is sold at the supermarket and it is advertised on television, the automatic message that derives from it is the following: it's good! Rather, the greater the advertising, the greater the sense of comfort and the perception of safety for the consumer that will have more security perception, which determines the increase of product sales.

Everyone knows how important the proper diet is: the problem is that very few know what is on the market. Sometimes unhealthy food is advertised as such also from experts in the field and, in the long period, can cause damages.

Unfortunately, there are a lots of disorders! Our body sends out signals constantly: intestinal discomfort, heartburn, abdominal swelling, constipation, headaches, various pains, often accompanied by weight gain or increased waist circumference.

Many people no longer notice the worsening of their wellness, and tend to consider all this as "normal" and due to our daily routine: work, stress, and ageing, neglecting to consider the reality.

Awareness as the Basis for Change

Each one of us, when approaching a dish, should be asking:

What food am I eating? Where does it come from? How was it prepared? What was it added with? We could add an infinity of questions. However, if we answer only a half of these, probably our food choices would change radically.

Your health is in your hands and it depends on your choices. Don't put off till tomorrow what you can do today!

Stop reflecting on all this and trying to implement a change will start the "turning point" of your life. Yes, because, turning thoughts into actions has a much higher value than you can imagine: step by step you can turn around the world, but if you stay still and keep procrastinating, you won't go anywhere! Asking yourself a series of questions represents the first step for what I call 'awareness'.

Think of something without acting like you're not being aware. When you start to act, your life surely will start to change.

Summary

- Many metabolic pathologies are related to nutrition.

- Processed food creates addiction.

- Awareness is necessary if you are looking for a change

- Turn your thoughts into actions.

The Meaning Of Weight Gain

In my view today only few people have a clear idea of what an increase in weight means.

The increase of weight is not just determined by a calorie increased intake, but is mostly due to poor efficiency of the body in metabolizing correctly the intake nutrients, clearly "clogged" by junk food, that makes it lose its potential and effectiveness.

My HND program will help you understand that the amount of calories must always be associated with the nutritional quality of food. Eating high quality food guarantees the introduction of vitamins, minerals, fiber and antioxidants. These are essential elements for our body, all very important for different aspects and functions, as well as for the regulation of numerous steps of metabolism. Therefore, the increase of weight is due to a low quality nutrition and, consequently, getting fat means mostly putting your own health at risk, as unhealthy food is one of the main causes of metabolic diseases. [2,3,4]

Body Composition and Metabolism

In the bi-compartmental model the body composition is divided into fat mass and lean mass.

The fat mass is composed mainly of fat (with low percentage of water), the lean mass is composed of everything else, so it is not just muscle, as probably many believe, but also water, tissues, bones, minerals and glycogen. [8,9,10]

In this case water is about 60% of the total body weight. This rate will be a little lower in women or in overweight people as in breasts and hips the percentage of fat increases. Thus, almost all the lean mass is made of water (obviously muscle cells included). [11]

Remember this crucial concept:

"When losing liquids, you certainly lose weight, obviously, but you are losing almost exclusively lean mass because, as explained above, the fat mass contains just small traces of water!"

Now onto defining the concept of metabolism:

Metabolism is, by definition, the set of synthesis reactions or degradations that take place in our body, in order to determine its growth, maintenance or renewal.

In other words, when we introduce food, our body will break it down in order to get energy necessary to carry out its functions, on one side, and rejecting elements on the other side, which will then be eliminated by our digestive organs (liver and kidney especially).

Returning to the previous discussion, it is useful to remember that the metabolically active cells, are therefore directly involved in metabolic processes, and part of the lean mass composed of about 95% of water.

Losing Weight and Low-Calorie Diets

Now that we have broadly explained the composition of the human body and how it works, let us now consider what losing weight consists of.

Given that, during our daily activities, most of which don't usually include physical exercise, our body prefers the use of fats as a main source of energy, although, it is always important to remember that the nervous system and the main organs use exclusively sugars for their "functioning". [12,13,14]

Summary:

Conditions of rest: Fats 80%; Sugars 20%

Things change with physical activity or general movement, where the consumption of sugars gradually increases even up to almost 100% of the total energy expenditure, under effort conditions at high intensity. [13]

Also, at the beginning of each activity (for example, we are seated and we stand up, we climb the stairs, we walk, etc.) our consumption will be composed, in those fractions of time, predominantly from sugars.

Baseline routine conditions: Fats 60%; Sugars 40%

Physical activity (average workout/high intensity): Fats 20%; Sugars 80%

How many calories do we consume? And, especially, how much fat?

We must consider that one kg of fat corresponds to a value that is around 7000 Kcal because the fat mass always has just a little fraction of water inside.

Consequently, restrictive diets, often called miraculous by those promoting them, are nothing more than pure illusion for those that, often disheartened, rely on the guru in charge hoping for a miracle: failure is assured!

Here's an example:

Let's say that Mrs. Pina, a 50-year-old sedentary and overweight woman, seeing herself as fat, decides to rely on her new guru who irresponsibly, with limited information as to her lifestyle and body composition, tells her she needs to lose 10 kg per month.

10 kg = 70000 Kcal.

Mrs. Pina, sedentary and with a little muscle mass, will have a daily consumption of roughly 1500/1600 Kcal

Hence: 1600 x 30 (days) = 48.000 Kcal

Simply put, if Mrs. Pina does not eat anything for a month, she can burn about 50 thousand calories, certainly not the 70 thousand suggested!

So even without eating anything she won't meet her goal!

Surely many overweight and/or obese people, have managed to lose ten kgs or more in a single month, but as already explained, that weight did not only belong to the fat mass, but probably, for the most part was constituted by liquids, then lean mass, since, as already stated, water is contained almost exclusively in lean cells.

It is true that a part of liquids is extracellular, or stagnation created by the overweight and bad habits, but a good fraction consists of "good" or intracellular liquid .

Very restrictive or unbalanced diets (for example high protein diets, of which we will be discussing in depth later), or low-calorie diets, lead to a state of semi-fasting.

In these circumstances, the body goes into "starvation mode", saving fat and using energy provided by muscle tissues (the proteins present in the muscles are degraded entering in the Krebs cycle or metabolic mill, in order to obtain vital sugars for metabolic functions mentioned above).

Key Point

If you follow low-calorie, unbalanced or otherwise restrictive diets, you are going to remove mainly water, therefore lean mass, generally muscle and metabolic mass, resulting in a less tonic body, a higher percentage of fat and able to "burn" less than before!

How Weight Loss Works

As explained above, "abnormal" conditions are always perceived as negative by the body, which then responds in a way to defend itself and offset the damage created: ***one must understand that our body is programmed to survive not to be "nice".***

Under conditions of food restriction, the body is activated and tries to maintain its energy reserves, eliminating those elements of lean mass, mainly muscle mass or metabolic mass, not only because they are considered less useful, but especially because of high energy consumption (adipose cells constitute an energy reserve, so they do not have a particularly active metabolism).

Let's take a simple example

If you had little fuel in the car, what would you do? A: accelerate and consume more? , B: drive slowly to make more efficient use of the fuel remaining?

Logic would dictate the answer is B. In fact, your body is programmed first and foremost for survival.

Summary:

"The body is programmed to survive, which is why in a food restricted condition energy saving and compensation mechanisms are activated." Once we understand this, it is easy to comprehend that the body will ultimately proceed with the elimination of fat, only if fed properly and in the best physical efficiency.

To explain further:

If we look at the human body depicted in anatomy or other science books, we never see them misshapen and with a belly! Normally, the model shown is the homo sapiens sapiens, well balanced, with good muscle tone and low fat mass.

Therefore, excess fat is not a natural component of the human body. Consequently, in conditions of good nutrition, muscle and metabolic mass will be restored and excess fat released. On a scientific level: when we are fed well , the fuel consumed at rest is mostly fat, so it will be the one to be eliminated if we have enough energy provided by the sugars needed to make our muscles, organs and nervous system work perfectly.

Listening To Yourself Is Fundamental

— On the other hand, if we listen to ourselves more mindfully, we are able to understand the different signals that our body sends. If we are hungry or have a feeling of hunger, it means one of these two things: We are either eating less, or we are eating badly.

Hunger is an alert and a defence mechanism, and is the only indication that our body sends out to let us understand that we are acting wrong:

"Do not bother to figure out how many calories you need, your body will make you aware of that; seek only to provide the right food, with high nutritional power, essential for, and compatible with our body!"

High Protein Diets

Most nutritional programs in vogue in recent years are certainly high-protein protocols, with many different names, but they all have essentially the same features: an excess of daily protein intake.

High-protein diets began to appear in the United States in the 70's with the Atkins diet, created by a renowned cardiologist, Robert Atkins.

Note that Dr. Atkins died in 2003 from obesity related conditions and apparently with heart problems as well.

Consistency is crucial: it is a contradiction to follow a weight loss diet, if it is prescribed by an obese nutritionist!

What do high-protein diets offer, and why are they followed? In short: "the promise of a fast and rapid weight loss by eating all that you want".

A real dream?

High-protein diets provide animal proteins almost exclusively (without considering that, as outlined below, proteins are everywhere, especially in the plant world).

Meat and fish are driven by the market (of course for economic interests), as well as all restaurants, from the cheapest to the most luxurious. They offer a variety of preparations and are easily available when you are dining out. People can eat them anywhere, with no problem and no restrictions and they can even lose weight! Fantastic!

Does It Really Work?

Rapid satiety and moderate caloric intake are surely points in favor, but the reason is easily explained: there are not many alternatives for breakfast, lunch, dinner and snacks if you do not eat meat, fish (mainly chicken breast and tuna), egg whites in large quantities and sometimes cheese without introducing other foods except some vegetables.

After a few weeks, the most obvious manifestation is a sense of nausea during meals, probably aggravated by the toxic effects of this food, which leads essentially to two conditions:

- Quit the diet

- Reduce the introduced food quantity (until gradually quitting the diet).

Failure is almost always determined by:

- Shortage of sugar (the main fuel of our body, especially in moderately intense physical exercise conditions).

- Shortage of essential micronutrients such as vitamins, minerals and antioxidants in general but also fiber.

Common Side Effects

- Constipation

- Gastrointestinal Discomfort And Burns

- Headache

- Bad Breath And Perspiration

- Energy Deficiency And General Fatigue

- Nausea

- Altered Blood Tests (When Dieting For An Extended Time)

These are just some of the most common symptoms; there are others, which can progress into various pathologies, that obviously do not outbreak immediately and are hardly ever associated to the concept of a wrong nutrition.

I would argue that:

"Whatever diet you decide to follow, if you have side effects, especially in the long term, it means that it is not healthy for your body."

"The ideal diet is the one that supports your mental and physical condition, without creating any kind of problem, but only benefits."

Weight Loss, But Loss of Lean Body Mass

The high protein diet usually becomes a low-calorie diet because after the first few days, the sense of nausea (due to the consumption of unhealthy and highly acidifying foods), and the monotony due to few suggested alternatives will cause you to eat less, possibly resulting in a substantial advantage on the weight scale and, I would add, only on this!

In fact, in order to eliminate the nitrogenous waste, the protein metabolism requires, through its processes, high quantity of water; the exact opposite of glucose metabolism in which the opposite happens (glycogen is linked to water).

By introducing very low values of carbohydrates, the body rapidly depletes its glycogen reserve (and thus also the watery part linked to it) in addition to using much more water, necessary to metabolize the disproportionate intake of proteins.

Consequently, besides the weight loss itself, due to a low-protein diet, a depletion of water contained in muscle tissues also occurs.

The resulting nutritional imbalance cannot bring the body to preserve its muscle mass, nor to increase it, as we very often hear!

Note that IGF1, the strongest anabolic hormone, as well as insulin, are routinely produced by our body, provided there are good nutritional conditions and when taking in the right amount of carbohydrates. [15]

For muscle growth, you must first perform workouts aimed at growth and carefully planned (possibly by professionals), and secondly have a balanced caloric intake adequate to physical commitments.

In summary: a good weight loss is achieved, but this loss is linked to that of water, then lean mass, with a good portion of the muscle mass.

Here's why losing weight does not mean becoming thinner!

It is rather the opposite, you are not going to tone up, especially in the absence of training as well as exposing the body to severe stress and metabolically dangerous situations.

Risk of a High Protein Diet

Here are the biggest risks for our body when following a high-protein diet:

- *Increase of uric acids:* the danger goes from articular pains to an increase of blood pressure, renal colic in association with the main metabolic diseases, such as diabetes and some tumor formation.

- *Change of the acid-base balance*: large protein loads lead to an excess of acidity due to protein oxidation (particularly the methionine and cysteine amino acids), and then to a compensation of our body thanks to calcium ions, "subtracted" from the bone mass (therefore also long-term skeletal risks with probable accompanying pathologies, osteoporosis in particular).

- *Kidney and liver overload*: these are the organs most affected by the protein metabolism.

- *Glycogen depletion.*

- *Loss of lean mass.*

- *Electrolyte imbalance and consequent risk of increased blood pressure*: not only the uric acid crystals are responsible, but also the large amount of sodium conveyed by foods containing animal proteins, aggravated by the non-compensation of other electrolytes, especially potassium for fresh fruit deficiency.

— *Increase of cardiovascular risk:* due to both the increase of pressure and uric acid, and the increase of cholesterol and saturated fat levels provided by animal products.

These are just the major consequences affecting the body subjected to a high-protein diet.

Unfortunately, I believe that long-term damage has been neither expected nor quantified yet: the truth is that if a particular diet can lead to these consequences in the short term, certainly it will only get worse in the long term!

Proteins and Physical Activity, a Look at Requirements

This applies to athletes, but there's an interesting aspect that concerns the protein requirement.

According to the SINU (Italian Society of Human Nutrition) through its LARN Report (Nutrition Intake Levels), the recommended intake levels for the Italian population are quite similar to the rest of the Western population (Europe and US). The protein requirement is approximately 0,8 g per kg of body weight; slightly increasing for subjects who do heavy work and advanced athletes with at least 15 hours of activities per week, where the value can increase to 1,5 max 1,8g per kg. For people who train 2 or 3 times per week without reaching the 5-6 hours of comprehensive training, the requirements are almost the same as those of sedentary individuals. [16]

These are studies that can be considered reliable as they are evaluated by measurements of nitrogen eliminated from the body, leaving little doubt as to the results.

On the other hand, I believe that a healthy body, fed correctly, does not require a high level of cellular "destruction" and does not have special requirements or need of spare parts as it's commonly argued (without valid documentation). In my opinion, it is more about marketing policies rather than science.

Athletes with a high competitive commitment, just need a slight protein increase, which is still covered by increased caloric intake (a 3000 Kcal/day diet doubles the intake of protein if compared to a 1500 Kcal/day diet), which does not justify any supplement.

Insights: Marketing and Proteins

We know that the profit of this big business is substantial, with very high yields (considered the cost/production ratio); moreover, it is difficult to eradicate the idea of 'necessity' instilled in our minds by manufacturers and by mass media in general.

What we need to question is the alleged miraculous effect of proteins that can help and maintain muscle growth as well as weight loss and good health condition, while the evidence (not only science) disproves this.

These days, the numbers of those overweight and suffering from obesity are concerning and as we know they are related to far more serious consequences such as severe metabolic problems.

These issues depend on the lifestyle and diet in general, and among the causes, include foods that are commonly defined as protein.

The marketing started from food and industrial farms, ending up with the market of supplements, of which we will discuss later.

What I would emphasize is the understanding that business and marketing are generally inversely proportional to the health conditions.

After understanding the steps related to weight loss, it is necessary on your part to build your own awareness, distance yourself from confusing trends, focus on health, and on the paths needed to achieve it.

Human Anatomy: The Great Luminaries Speak

Before describing the HND method, it is important to understand some basic notions of biology and human anatomy.

Numerous statement have been made around these matters, although sometimes inaccurate.

I believe it is simplistic to synthesize an era that lasted hundreds of years with sweeping statements such as that man was a hunter or rather an omnivore, etc. However, I would not concentrate too much on the past, since it no longer exists and has little relationship to modern humans.

It is like trying to understand how a particular application of my new Smartphone works and then studying the operations of a telephone booth from the 80s. Everything is different, everything has evolved (for better or for worse), so you need to have more current references, then make an analysis of the reality that we have available, without getting lost in discussions overcome by the evolutionary process.

We begin by saying that man has about 99.5% of genetic material in common with the chimpanzee, (the closest species to the human race). Accordingly, we will refer to how these primates eat. The food usually consumed by a Chimpanzee is mainly fruit, (hence, they are commonly referred to as "frugivorous ") then leaves, berries, seeds and shrubs, sometimes few-insects or eggs (rarely).

Now, looking at the human anatomy, we can make some observations:

MOUTH: we have a dentition with wide incisors, molars and flat premolars, small canines, accompanied by an ability to chew (and therefore the jaw that moves in multiple directions) with abundant salivation, able to mix and homogenize the food well before transferring it to the next stages.

Observations: anatomically speaking, humans can be considered as frugivorous (the carnivore has fixed jaws, rips and does not chew, large and sharp canines, small incisors, very little production of saliva and swallows bites without chewing).

GASTROINTESTINAL SYSTEM: Man has a long, narrow, spongy intestine with bends and curvatures, also has a reduced amount of acidic juices, with the absence of the uricase enzyme (fundamental to disrupt the uric acid produced by the protein metabolism).

Observations: as far as the complex digestive tract, we reflect in full the frugivorous species: carnivores have short intestines, devoid of curves and essentially smooth, in order to facilitate a rapid digestion with a consequent expulsion of rotting substances.

Carnivores have a hydrochloric acid value about 10 times higher than human's, in such a way as to degrade large protein quantities. They also have the uricase enzyme, which allows them to digest 30g. of uric acid produced by the metabolism of each kg of animal protein ingested.

OTHER CHARACTERISTICS: Human blood has a pH of 7.3/7.5, alkaline; a carnivore around 6 (depending on the species), so decidedly acidic, whereby the alkaline foods (fruits and vegetables in particular), are certainly more compatible with the human anatomical features (only the quantity of 30g. of protein would lead to acidification in the blood, if there were not "buffer" systems to take action).

The human immune system, as demonstrated by Kouchakoff, operates with a high leukocyte response to the introduction of meals containing meat or animal proteins in general, recognizing them as "enemies". [17]

Breast milk has very little protein, almost comparable to fruit, unlike milk of other animals, especially carnivores, whose value is much higher (dogs and cats have 30 and 40% of protein, respectively).

Observations: we say that we have very little in common with carnivores and the evidence is clear: we have the hands to collect and no claws to hunt and kill. Our instinct is not homicidal.

How many of you would approach a carcass to eat it and when I say eat it I mean like the carnivores, organs bitten with the body still in agony (the carnivores feed on blood and organs not rotting carcasses).

Do you feel more attracted to a beautiful, colourful fruit or to slaughtering the body of a poor beast? And above all: how many of you would dare to do it?

The statements of great luminaries

I close this "anatomical" talk with the statements of the father, founder of comparative anatomy, Georges Cuvier (1769-1832) and other great luminaries.

Thanks to Cuvier's studies, it has been possible to reconstruct, step by step, some extinct species.

"The Comparative Anatomy teaches us that humans resemble frugivorous animals in every detail and not at all carnivores... Only by disguising dead flesh, made more tender by culinary techniques, it is possible for humans to chew and digest it, just so the sight of raw and bloody meat does not arouse horror and disgust ".

Richard Owen, naturalist (1804-1892):

A) The anthropoids and all quadrumanes eat fruit, seeds and other juicy vegetable matter. The close analogy between the structure of animals and that of man clearly demonstrates their natural frugivourism.

B) The apes, whose dentition is almost equal to that of man, live mainly on fruit, nuts and other similar variety for consistency, flavor and nutritional value processed by the plant world. The profound similarity between the teeth of quadrumanes and those of men shows that man was originally adapted to eat fruit from the trees in Paradise.

Dr. Richard Lane, anatomist:

"Comparative anatomy proves that human dentition is totally frugivorous, and this is confirmed by paleo-zoological studies with documented data going back millions of years."

Carolus Linnaeus, botanist (1707-1778):

"Fruit is the most suitable food to man's mouth, stomach and hands, designed to collect and eat fruit. And even if mankind at some point in its history adopted omnivorous habits, millions of years of "omnivourism" have not changed the anatomy and physiology of his body."

HND: HEALTHY NATURAL DIET

Introduction
The Importance of Awareness

After this extensive but necessary introduction, we have come to the crucial part of this book, and we are going to describe the diet that has the potential to change your life.

The HND is a universal nutritional program suitable for anyone in any physical condition.

On these grounds alone, we can argue that HND is a winning solution.

More than a simple dietary protocol, HND, promotes a shift in lifestyle, enabling you to easily make changes to your way of living, thinking, and reasoning, mainly in your relationship with food and consequently, on your overall health.

I'm talking about changes because if a person learns about the metabolism of certain principles, it is practically impossible to go back. The new habits become definitive (i.e., think about your driving skills: once you have learned how to drive, it's impossible for you to 'unlearn' it).

These changes must come from the inside, in which case the benefits will affect to the whole body.

Therefore, you cannot eat and live according to HND if you don't fully understand what this method really is.

If we merely follow HND without this understanding, we will keep making the same mistakes that will ultimately result in yet another failed attempt at improving our quality of life.

As I have often underlined, human beings are a combination of mind, body and spirit, and whatever you do, it is essential to first understand it and then internalize it so it becomes who you are.

If you consider any activity or interest in an isolated manner, you will hardly be able to implement it effectively and satisfactorily.

For example, It is useless to read a book if you do not love reading: in a few days you set that book aside; or, ask a person to train if he doesn't have the passion for the sport: one might also join a gym, driven by the initial enthusiasm but most likely will soon resume the same old habits.

Finally, whatever you decide to do, you have to do it with all your being. Also, you need to understand what you are doing: desires, excitement, easy enthusiasm may be good intentions, but serve no purpose, except perhaps bring more disappointment for being unable to achieve those accomplishments.

This is why I would suggest you to think carefully about what I am proposing, otherwise it becomes useless to try, because it will not help you reach your goals. Attempts made at random, as if to say "let me give this a try and then I'll see" are unnecessary and disastrous.

I have personally experienced several times having an interest in a hobby or a sport that had initially impressed me, but soon after, I had no incentive to continue.

There's nothing bad or wrong with that, it's just a fact!

After all, devoting yourself to something and doing it well takes time, passion and perseverance! It is said that man's attention can only be focused on one goal at a time: I think that is actually true!

These days, we are "forced" to meet more commitments at the same time (family, work, our personal interests), but in the long run it becomes difficult to control everything perfectly, so you do what you can!

I don't believe in people who seek external motivation or help from others, as if to say: "Come on let's do it together."

This is because desire and motivation should start from the inside: this is the only way to build up all of the energy needed to pursue something. Those who struggle for help from the outside will achieve little because in reality, all you're going to get, depends solely upon you.

Health is important and valuable, so mine is an invitation to understand this so as to be ready and determined for a definitive change: if you really want to achieve well-being, know that there is a way and you can do it, but you need awareness first and foremost

Difficulties and fear of change

The classic answer that I hear from friends, colleagues or patients, is: "We've always done that!" "We've always eaten this way!".

It is important to understand the following, as it applies not only in the field of Dietology, but life in general.

To define it you might say: *fear of change.*

We all have created our own daily routine, all around us people doing pretty much the same things; consequently, this means that it is correct and necessary to do so.

If all restaurants offer the same menu, if TV, radio or newspapers give the same news, if nutrition experts recommend that kind of food, or they consider a certain product as "normal " or, simply to limit, (which happens at a general level in the food industry), it means that actually everything else is wrong, risky, and could lead to dangerous consequences.

Accordingly, changing the type of one's diet could mean not only to create instability in our daily life, which could be a laborious process, both at a family and social level, but it would also mean having to "conflict" with important institutions supporting completely different theories.

The difficulty of change, almost always accompanied with dissenting opinions, can be discouraging to even those with the best intentions for positive lifestyle changes. Therefore, most people find it easier to simply follow the status quo of long held beliefs regardless of its effectiveness in improving their health and welfare over the long term.

Open-Minded and Inclined to Change

How many times have I heard "Now, what do I eat?" Or "What will I do?" "How will I act at a dinner with friends or when I invite someone home?"

Often, after less than a week, the most common thoughts are: "No, I can't do it, it's too hard, it's not for me!".

Although we are talking about fairly simple steps, when you are trapped in your comfort zone, they become insurmountable obstacles.

Our daily life teaches us that in order to feel better, to be able to improve and evolve, it is necessary to change and thus adapt ourselves to a new system.

Take for example, mobile phones: not long ago, it would have been unthinkable to write a text message; now practically everything is done with a phone, and even the most reluctant have had to adapt themselves to keep up with the times.

The same thing is happening with nutrition: when several years ago I suggested my patients to eliminate meat from their diet, I was regarded as an extremist; now those people are no longer eating meat or have considerably reduced their intake, as they have become aware of the risks that it produces.

As a result, in a few years since, this habit has become quite common, so much so that today it is considered "normal" choosing to not eat meat.

However, it is important to understand that everything is "normal" only when the system accepts it: years ago, in order to learn about dangers linked to meat consumption, it was necessary to obtain information from the world's remote sources of "mass media" and the nutrition and health institutions in general.

As I previously mentioned, people are afraid of changes, afraid to jeopardize their habits and their knowledge.

If, like me, you have a thirst for knowledge or have any doubts, or you are simply eager to understand, you'll probably have to get away from the "safety" of everyday life.

The choice is hard, because it involves not only reconsidering our daily routine, but may very well also call into question the whole of our existence.

Thus, I will not tell you to choose: to choose requires awareness.

Listen to your inner voice with an open mind and ready to change. Everything else will be a natural consequence.

What is wellness?

It is correct to ask ourselves this question, although it doesn't have such an obvious answer. We each have our own concept of wellness

According to the HND method, the 'wellness' term is synonymous with harmony, clarity, and performance. This creates an efficiency that encompasses the whole of our mind, body and spirit.

That's why you cannot just focus on the physical aspect, because other crucial characteristics of human nature would be excluded.

Depression, eating disorders, and many other problems arise mainly as a mind-body dissonance. There is no harmony, and when you create a duality in something which needs to stand united, it inevitably creates conflict.

Of course, in this book, more space will be devoted to the field of nutrition and physical activity, but it is important to understand that in order to change.

"Mens Sana in Corpore Sano", the famous quote by Decimo Giunio Giovenale, a great roman poet: if it's still valid after almost two thousand years, there must be a reason!

Being in harmony with what is the true nature of man is the crucial prerequisite to reach a state of well-being.

The Meaning of HND

Before describing the HND method, it is right to explain the origin and the meaning.

The most significative letter of this acronym is definitely the N (natural), H (healthy) is a consequence of N, and D (diet) because it is a diet which, I recall, is a word that derives from the Greek and means "life style" So, again, the diet is not a piece of paper with some recommendations , but according to my definition:

"A guideline on how to behave in terms of nutrition, physical activity and lifestyle in order to achieve the greatest state of psycho-physical well-being"

In summary, the best definition is *HND method.*

Why nature?

In HND, N stands for Natural so 'in a natural way'. I chose this term because I believe that nature should be part of any diet plan.

Nature has always established a balance, especially at a global level, for which, thanks to it, hundreds of ecosystems are able to exist in harmony with each other.

"Those who eat what nature offers, will hardly ever face problems."

Animal species eating plants, grass or fruit do not get fat, obese, they never have high cholesterol, diabetes or die from arteriosclerosis and cancer

Nature is perfect, animals do not need to lose their nature to provide their own food: for example, we will never see a cow eating a lion!

A trivial example, but with the intent to make you think.

Understandably, for logistic reasons, convenience or other issues, one is often forced to make convenient choices, but nowadays unfortunately, we have lost a lot of relations with the natural world.

"Who I am, what relationship I have within this ecosystem, what is my true essence": maybe just few people question themselves about these topics.

We got to the point of analysing our genes in order to understand the causes of obesity and diseases related to it, but a clear solution is under everybody's eyes, although too often ignored due to private interests, poor knowledge and convenience.

The HND Diet (Healthy Natural Diet)

So that it can be better understood, first I will explain the HND model and its physical aspects. Then we will delve into what it means to live and eat according to the HND program. Eating within the HND program is simple, practical and fast, as it is not necessary to find special foods, use special preparations or buy supplements.

HND respects geographical areas and the seasonality of foods, so you can eat and adapt the method wherever you are located.

Obviously, if you travel to Antarctica it will be more difficult to find certain products. However, with the progress we have achieved in transportation, it is not impossible to follow the instructions, although not 100% (this applies to any other diet as well).

HND presents few difficulties, but it still requires the desire to experiment and some creativity on your part. Doing this will help you to become even more invested and thrilled at how nutrition can give you the chance to invent new dishes. You need to be fully committed if you wish to succeed in what you do!

In fact, once you acquire your culinary skills, you can create so many recipes thanks to the use of the HND method.

HND and Vegan Model

HND is a total vegetable diet, which excludes animal products, processed foods, and industrial contamination.

However, it would be simplistic to consider the HND method as just a "vegan" diet.

HND and veganism are two different concepts. In fact:

"Everything that is healthy is also vegan, but not vice versa"

Let us better explain this point starting from the definition of veganism.

Vegans are those individuals that, for ethical and philosophical reasons, where possible and feasible, follow a lifestyle consisting in the refusal of all animal products and refrain from all practices connected to the exploitation of animals.

This definition does not include the concept of "healthy nutrition".

Proper nutrition is a science that must be studied in-depth and properly.

To understand the nutritional principles, you need to refer to medical and scientific matters, particularly chemistry and biochemistry.

Without a scientific basis, it is difficult to understand the effect that food has on the human body.

In recent times, emerging and growing businesses in this field, also promoted by mass media, have given rise to some confusion.

Dietology is now treated with very little care, often manipulated by non-professionals.

This is also why the concept of "vegan diet = healthy diet" has become so popular.

Once established, this belief has encouraged food and supplement producers to take advantage of the growing demand for healthy products, in the interest of high profits and to the detriment of the now even more confused consumers. We are currently observing:

- Veganism for ethical reasons

- Veganism for fashion

- People who eat poorly or who reject traditional medicine believing that eating vegan means taking good care of themselves.

— People who attack the vegan movement for various and groundless reasons.

Let's clarify the concept of healthy nutrition.

1. **Veganism Is an Ethical Concept,** not a trend. Those who become vegans make this choice because they respect animals. In my opinion this is right: bioethics come first and foremost, and all living beings have equal rights on the earth. But this has nothing to do with the nutritional and scientific principles previously mentioned (true vegans do not necessarily care if what they do is nutritionally healthy). As an example: a Muslim who observes Ramadan doesn't have the goal to lose weight!

2. **Eating Vegan Does Not Mean Eating Healthy**: Avoiding animal products is healthier and more compatible with human nutrition and can prevent major metabolic diseases. However, an animal- protein free diet is not necessarily a healthy diet. It is important to remember that industrial sugars and white flours are the real enemies (the latter are basically a concentration of sugar and modified gluten), also industrial sweeteners, thickeners, colorings, preservatives or stabilizers, even though not derived from animals, are very harmful for our body. We need to consider that some methods of preparation or food processing do not provide active principles to our body, and they often damage it (for example oil cooking). Consequently, it is clear that being vegan it is not enough to eat healthy.

3. **The Vegan Business Is Misleading, Sometimes Harmful to Health:** The food industry is obviously interested in marketing food and does not really care about consumers'

health. They produce meat substitutes or other foods devoid of animal products but rich in sugars, vegetable oils and thickeners. After all, the population is accustomed to poor nutritional habits. Therefore, in order to create a product with good organoleptic properties, it is necessary to add "tasty," although unhealthy substances.

4. **One Cannot Expect A 100% Healthy Diet Without Excluding Animal Products**. Logically, for the aforementioned reasons regarding the human anatomy and its compatible foods, it is unlikely to think about having perfect health or simply the maximum benefit and performance from your body if you continue to eat animal foods.

Avoid Unnecessary Classifications: Many like to "label" people. Personally, I do not think it's correct, because humans are so complex and fascinating that it would be simplistic to define them with a simple adjective.

The Nutritional Power of Food

To explain the cornerstone of the HND system, I will give a small example: Let's take a fresh orange, just harvested, an orange juice and a fruit juice from the supermarket. All three have the same calories, but will the sense of satiety that you feel after consumption be the same?

Probably what makes you feel better and more satisfied is the whole orange, potentially more nutritious than the other two choices.

Hence the concept of what I call the *nutritional power* of food.

Definition

The nutritional power of food is the ability of a particular food to provide a sense of wellness and satiety to our body.

The higher the nutritional value, the higher the resulting sense of well-being.

The Quality Is Fundamental

As mentioned earlier, the Healthy Natural Diet gives more importance to the quality of food rather than the calories.

Basically, you need to consume foods with high nutritional value meaning those natural foods able to provide a considerable amount of nutrients in terms of vitamins, minerals, phytochemicals and antioxidants because they have undergone very little, if any, processing.

Only by consuming natural foods, can we satisfy our needs, providing the body with a large amount of "clean" energy without the extra effort of eliminating unnecessary waste and toxins capable of irreparably modifying our physical, metabolic and genetic structure.

Organics

The HND program encourages you to consume seasonal, non-contaminated products. So, unless you have your own garden, or you have reliable local farmers, in supermarkets buy organic.

What is the meaning of organic farming?

Organic farming does not use synthetic chemicals such as fertilizers, herbicides, fungicides, insecticides and pesticides in general, nor GMOs (genetically modified organisms).

It ensures crop rotation, by avoiding the cultivation of the same plant on the same soil for several consecutive seasons. This procedure prevents parasites from finding favorable environments and proliferating. Moreover, the nutrients present in the soil are exploited less intensively.

For safe production, it is necessary to have trees or hedges around the farm in order to provide a welcome atmosphere to the pests' predators and acts as a physical barrier to possible external pollution.

Organic farming requires the simultaneous cultivation of different plants that in synergy eliminate parasites from each other.

Natural fertilizers, such as manure and other composted organic substances, are used in organic farming. If necessary, other natural substances derived from plants, animals or minerals, authorized by the EC Regulation (highlighted exhaustively in a separated list) can be used to protect crops.

Organic products are labelled as such, easily recognizable, provided that the producer was declared compliant to the specific regulations by competent authorities.

Understandably, organic farming is not easily accessible to all those who wish to ensure compliance, safety and quality in food; in some cases, companies have been indicted for fraud due to selling organic products where there weren't any; and other companies have obtained the "organic" trademark without having met the requirements.

From my point of view, regulations and supervision are strict in many states, so it is not correct to generalize, or think that everything is exclusively business.

For your greater safety, you can use some precautions. Two in particular:

- Be aware and respect the seasonality of foods.

- Examine foods carefully: imperfections, dull colour, size, are all characteristics that help us distinguish natural food from processed food.

The Seasonality of Food

I consider seasonal foods to be essential in the Healthy Natural Diet and commonly referred to as 'live foods', mostly fruits and vegetables. These foods have high nutritional value, and because they are 'alive', decay rapidly after being harvested. They are high in vitamins, antioxidants and bio-available phytochemicals, so very important for our body. Packaged foods, as well as animal meat, pre-cooked foods and ready to eat meals, do not have a high nutritional power, and are not really compatible with the human body.

Below, is a very interesting table showing the seasons of fruit and vegetable production (in Italy and in most of the states of the Mediterranean basin).

Vegetables	Jan	Feb	Mar	Apr	May	Jun	Jul	Aug	Sept	Oct	Nov	Dec
Garlic	X	X	X	X	X	X	X	X	X	X	X	X
Asparagus				X	X	X						
Beets	X	X	X	X	X	X	X	X	X	X	X	X
Artichokes	X	X	X	X	X	X					X	X
Thistle	X										X	X
Carrots	X	X	X	X	X	X	X	X	X	X	X	X
Cauliflower	X	X	X	X	X	X				X	X	X
Chicory	X	X	X	X					X	X	X	X
Onions	X	X	X	X	X	X	X	X	X	X	X	X
Green Beans				X	X	X	X	X	X	X		
Fava Beans				X	X							
Fennels	X	X	X	X					X	X	X	X
Lettuce				X	X	X	X	X	X	X		
Aubergines						X	X	X	X	X	X	
Potatoes	X	X	X	X	X	X	X	X	X	X	X	X
Peppers						X	X	X	X	X	X	
Peas				X	X	X	X					
Tomatoes						X	X	X	X	X		
Leek	X	X	X	X					X	X	X	X
Radicchio	X	X	X	X	X					X	X	X
Celery	X	X	X	X	X	X	X	X	X	X	X	X
Spinach	X	X	X	X					X	X	X	X
Cabbage	X	X	X	X	X	X	X	X	X	X	X	X
Zucchini				X	X	X	X	X	X	X	X	X

Fruits	Jan	Feb	Mar	Apr	May	Jun	Jul	Aug	Sept	Oct	Nov	Dec
Apricot						X	X					
Oranges	X	X	X	X	X				X	X	X	X
Persimmon											X	X
Chestnut										X	X	X
Cherries						X	X					
Clementine	X	X								X	X	X
Watermelons						X	X	X				
Strawberries				X	X	X						
Kiwi	X	X	X	X						X	X	X
Lemons	X	X	X	X	X	X	X	X	X	X	X	X
Apples	X	X	X	X	X	X	X	X	X	X	X	X

	1	2	3	4	5	6	7	8	9	10	11	12
Melons					X	X	X	X	X	X		
Pears	X	X	X	X	X	X	X	X	X	X	X	X
Peaches					X	X	X	X	X			
Plum						X	X	X				
Grapes							X	X	X	X	X	

Of course, seasonality is also valid for grains and legumes. Although they do not have the same nutritional value as fruits and vegetables, they have good nutritional properties. Seasonality means that in a natural and spontaneous way, the products tend to grow during certain periods, without the need for special human "aid".

This implies that they do not require any chemical treatment in order to facilitate production.

As a result, the product harvested is "clean" enough, and therefore healthy.

However, during the good season, some vegetables and fruits, as well as cereals or legumes, are subjected to chemical treatments in order to prevent parasitic attacks. Strawberries, for example, require numerous treatments, even during their growing and harvest season.

For this reason, you must be very careful, especially in supermarkets, where they often sell huge waxed strawberries, too "perfect" to be natural and free from contamination.

Whereas a wild strawberry, grown in your garden or in the undergrowth will certainly lose its good looks within a day!

In conclusion, it is not that difficult to distinguish quality products. To help you in your choices, refer to locals or small farmers, who often sell the products of their harvest to local markets. Visually analyze what you purchase and if you have any doubts, make other choices.

No one can guarantee 100% that you are buying a perfect product free of contamination, but paying attention to simple details allows you to move towards safer and healthier options.

Table: Pesticides In Fruits And Vegetables

High Concentration Of Pesticides	Low Concentration Of Pesticides
Apples	Avocado
Strawberries	Pineapple
Grapes	Cabbage
Celery	Onions
Peaches	Asparagus
Spinach	Mango
Peppers	Papaya
Nectarines	Kiwi
Cucumber	Aubergines
Tomatoes	Grapefruit
Peas	Cauliflower
Potatoes	Sweet Potatoes

Calories in the Healthy Natural Diet

As already mentioned earlier, calories are just one of the many elements in the HND method. They are certainly important, but not essential, and I would like to explain why.

If we consume only natural foods, compatible with the human structure and therefore easy to digest, with a minimum of waste content and free of leukocyte response, we will provide our body with high quality fuel.

If the quality of our food is good, we will not experience changes in the endocrine and hormones levels, primarily responsible for the senses of hunger and satiety.

Therefore, we do not need to pay attention to calories because the body, adjusting itself, does so automatically by promptly sending the satiety signals.

Do you believe that a body as complex as ours, capable of running numerous sophisticated functions simultaneously would not be able to tell us when and especially how much we need to eat?

Just like the mechanism of thirst: you do not need to understand when and how much to drink, because your body sends out signals when necessary.

Summary:

HND foods do not produce changes to the body, and so allow us to perceive hunger/satiety signals. Therefore, you don't need to worry about calories and only need pay attention to the quality of the food.

To be more precise:

I understand that starting a new diet can be difficult, especially in terms of sources of supply and intake quantity, but this will only affect the early stage. Each one of us that approaches the HND system, has his own specific psychological and physical conditions: some might have always eaten well enough, naturally interested in nutrition and inclined to physical activity, whilst others might have done exactly the opposite and therefore present a high degree of toxicity, along with all biological and receptive signals in disarray.

So, my advice to HND followers, is to define a general framework in order to gather precise information then proceed autonomously and ask for clarifications if doubts should arise.

Sense of Hunger: An Important Bell

When I mention "hunger", I refer to a mechanism that causes the body to ask for food and not hunger as food shortage (which, I believe, would be quite offensive towards those people struggling daily to survive starvation).

Hunger is a need as is thirst: if you are hungry you must eat, likewise, if you are thirsty, you must drink. Unfortunately, we tend to do the opposite of what the body expects us to do.

Through the years, I have seen so much in dietology: supplements, capsules, tablets, tricks of all kinds devised by the "gurus" of nutrition in order to mask this important signal.

While trying to stop a correct stimulus (though our body is hardly mistaken), no one thinks about the cause of that stimulus, in fact the most important thing is to ask ourselves why we get hungry.

The answer is simple. As we continue to eat incorrectly and provide our body with artificial and harmful substances, we become hungry for high calorie meals that are low in nutrients.

As a consequence, the hunger/satiety signals are chemically altered, creating major insulin and hormonal imbalances such as to literally off-balance our body. It is important to remember that the sense of satiety is affected not only by calories, but also by other key elements such as fiber or some essential micro-elements involved in various metabolic processes.

Eating "empty" calories means to noticeably prolong satiety. For example, how much ice cream can you eat before you feel satiated and satisfied? Maybe even more than a kilo which means introducing 3-4 thousand calories.

Try to consume the equivalent calories in fresh fruit if you can!

Once again, it is important to consider the nutritional power of food. Natural foods are complete, since, thanks to their rich composition of vitamins, minerals, fiber and bioavailable antioxidants that provide the body the essential elements that are necessary for the satiety processes.

Eating according to the HND model leads to a restored balance of hunger/satiety signals in our bodies.

No need to worry about how much you eat or to count calories, as it is the body, now fully functional, that will respond in an immediate way to satiety signals.

With HND you will finally discover positive feelings never felt before. We must not hold back from eating food nor strive to define what and when to eat to be satisfied without having to struggle every day with the scale!

Healthy Natural Diet Foods

The Healthy Natural Diet, as already explained, consists of only natural foods.

Obviously it is advisable, at least in the early stages, to be monitored by a professional, as not all start from the same physical conditioning, and especially don't all do the same job, the same degree of physical activity, nor lead the same lifestyle.

In general, we can summarize:

— Fruit (At Least 3 Times Per Day)

— Vegetables (At Least 2 Times Per Day)

— Tubers (1-2 Times Per Day)

— Whole Grains (1 Time Per Day)

— Herbaceous Plants (1 Time Per Day)

— Seeds (2 Times Per Day)

— Dried Fruit (3-5 Times Per Week)

— Legumes (4-5 Times Per Week)

It is important TO reaffirm that HND is a diet that respects nature and THE seasonality of food that provides eating mainly what the land of their environment offers.

In addition to being ethically sustainable, diets based on local and seasonal products, ensure nutrients in higher and in more bioavailable amounts.

For example, if you compare a freshly harvested ripe mango with an imported mango, picked unripe and that has undergone several treatments before reaching the final consumer, it is understandable that the nutritional power is completely different.

Main features of the Healthy Natural Diet foods

What follows is a general description of the specific foods, according to the Healthy Natural Diet.

I will not expand on this list because you can investigate further on specific books or by browsing the internet.

My intention is to briefly summarize the key characteristics of each family examined to assess its importance.

Fruit

Fruit is our most recommended fuel.

There are many varieties of fruit: from the aqueous fruits such as oranges, watermelon, melon, strawberries, kiwi, peach, to the more caloric and filling such as bananas, figs, khaki; from starchy fruits such as chestnuts to the oily ones such as coconut or the precious avocado.

There are fruits that have incredible nutritional properties, also known as superfruits such as pomegranate, pitaya, noni and mangosteen or other fruits that have a fabulous enzymatic capacity, very helpful for digestion, such as pineapples or papaya.

We have fruit with great nutritional power, such as red apples and others capable of restoring imbalances such as lemons.

Then berries, the fruits of the forest family, such as: black currant, raspberries, blackberries or blueberries, rich in antioxidants and phytochemicals with unique properties helpful for the cardiovascular and immune systems as well as eyes, spleen, liver and blood vessels.

This is only a small part of what the world of fruit is: an excellent food source for human beings.

By listing the properties of various fruits on the planet, I can say that, in the Healthy Natural Diet, no fruit need be avoided, as they all have vitamins, minerals and antioxidants essential to guarantee our health and long-term wellness. The more the variety of choices, the more the benefits, especially if they act in synergy between them.

As already mentioned, the instruction given is to respect the seasonality of fruit and especially the origin and growing areas.

It makes little sense to consume strawberries in winter or mangos in the Nordic countries. The taste changes considerably, as well as the nutritional properties.

Long distance transports imply harvesting fruits when still unripe: those fruits that do not ripen on the plant and often undergo chemical treatments to extend their conservation, have a decidedly inferior nutritional power.

The same happens if you do not respect the seasonality: when forgetting about this aspect, one is consuming fruit produced elsewhere.

Surely, at some latitudes, there are incredible advantages because you can also eat almost exclusively fruit; in other latitudes, however, it is more difficult due to adverse weather conditions.

The important thing is to make the most correct, and therefore healthier decisions: if we live in a Nordic country, for example, it will be more healthful eating an apple, though not directly produced there , rather than a banana.

Remember that fruit with shell such as the coconut is more protected and less contaminated than others, so also quite resistant to long trips.

Vegetables

Vegetables are, with fruit, the fundamental pillar of the Healthy Natural Diet.

As with fruits, there are many varieties, from leafy vegetables to greens.

They have no energy properties, but they are very useful for their purifying power: essential to provide the body with vitamins, minerals and antioxidants, as well as to supply a major source of fiber.

Vegetables have different colors and it is the color that often identifies the precious nutrients they contain.

In red vegetables (tomatoes, peppers) we distinguish, for example lycopene, a potent anticancer; beta carotene (carrots, squash, peppers) that exerts strong protection against free radicals and is characteristic of orange vegetables; chlorophyll, with its powerful, purifying and antioxidant action, is present in all green leaves (salads, spinach, chicory, endive, beets, celery). The blue-violet color (radicchio, aubergines, purple cabbage, beets, brussels sprouts), indicates the presence of anthocyanins, very precious antioxidants to prevent cancer, cardiovascular diseases and kidney-urinary tract diseases; the white color (cabbage, cauliflower, garlic, onion) ensures the presence of quercetin, a powerful anticancer.

All vegetables are recommended in the Healthy Natural Diet. You only need pay attention to product quality and, with regard to certain greens, the ripeness.

This applies in particular for tomatoes, peppers, and aubergines, but also for potatoes, which contain a substance, solanine, that can be toxic in small quantities.

This substance is reduced significantly with ripening, although it is better overdo it, and try to vary the consumption of vegetables in order to introduce all of the precious nutrients and phytochemicals, which are characteristic of each family.

Vegetables are crucial and, especially if eaten raw, help restore intestinal balance and all digestive processes.

Tubers and Roots

Generally tubers and roots have exceptional properties, so in the Healthy Natural Diet it is recommended to consume them regularly.

In this family, we can distinguish the tubers precisely such as: potatoes, red potatoes (or sweet potatoes), manioc, which are also an excellent source of important starches and highly bioavailable; then there are the real roots, whose properties are comparable to the vegetables. These include beets, daikon, Jerusalem artichokes, celeriac, and horseradish, but also ginger and turmeric.

The tubers are indicated as an excellent cereal substitute, indeed, in some ways they are preferable to them, as they are more digestible, with more nutritional properties and less subject to contamination processes.

In addition to starches, especially amylopectin (the most digestible and assimilable component of starch), they contain fiber, vitamins, potassium, magnesium, iron, calcium, flavonoids and anthocyanins. They have great antioxidant properties.

It is recommended to cook them before consumption.

However, roots should be eaten raw in order to fully assimilate the precious vitamins, minerals and antioxidants they contain.

You can of course also boil them and use them as ingredients for soups, purées and other preparations.

Their leaves, even if characterized by a strong and very sour taste, are rich in vitamins, minerals and other properties, so it's worth eating them with fresh lemon juice, or at least to make smoothies or soups.

My advice, obviously when you are sure of the origin, is to eat tubers after cooking and raw peeled roots in order to absorb all of the nutrients.

Insights: The Red Beet

The beetroot is a tuber with extraordinary properties that should always be on our tables, despite its particularly strong taste, especially if eaten raw, a little uninviting for palates accustomed to "industrial" foods.

It has a good amount of fiber, both soluble and insoluble, and it is important not only for satiating power, but especially for modulating the levels of sugar and cholesterol in the blood.

It is an important source of minerals, including iron, but also sodium, potassium, calcium, magnesium and iodine.

It contains B Vitamins, beta carotene and Vitamin C in abundance.

The beet is also a concentration of anthocyanins, precious antioxidants.

You can eat all of this tuber, including leaves and roots.

The advice is to consume raw or thinly sliced with lemon juice or in salads.

Great supplement for athletes

Beet roost turn out to be extraordinarily useful for athletes and sports activities in general, especially for endurance sport practitioners.

In the Healthy Natural Diet, I always suggest to this group of athletes, to make a juice or an extract of beetroot with two lemons in the morning when you wake up and right after a hard workout, to ensure balance in blood parameters, especially iron and hematocrit.

Grains

Cereals have always represented the basic element of human nutrition.

Without grains different populations would become extinct. This food plays an important role in the field of dietology, despite being classified, by many, as not always healthy for humans.

This is because it's usually not considered that processed products prepared with cereal derivatives have nothing to do with the natural product.

Brown rice in Asia, maize in South America, wheat, barley or spelt in Europe and in the Mediterranean basin, have always guaranteed nutrition and survival to their people, especially in cold periods or winter, when fruit and vegetables are scarce.

Grains, especially if high-quality, taken at the right times, in the right quantities and not mixed with other foods, are greatly tolerated by the body.

In the Healthy Natural Diet whole grain cereals are included exclusively, as they do not undergo chemical processes, hence, they do not lose their precious vitamins and minerals, especially in the external part of the grain named caryopsis.

Grains are rich in complex carbohydrates, but also in protein and fiber. They are important sources of B Vitamins, Vitamin E (contained in the small lipid portion of the wheat grain) and folic acid.

They are also excellent sources of minerals, including zinc, magnesium and selenium.

Among other cereals acceptable within the HND program are brown rice, barley, spelt, oats, maize and common wheat, of course, only if organic and therefore without industrial contamination or glyphosate and herbicide treatments.

Today, unfortunately, we tend to consider the 00 flours as being derived from wheat, neglecting to highlight that they come from intensive farming and industrial contaminating processes.

Respecting circadian cycles is fundamental in HND, so it is advisable to consume cereals mainly at lunch, and in small quantities in the evening.

Also, in order to avoid digestive problems, it is good to consume cereals in combination with vegetables, and possibly some seasonings like avocados, seeds or olive oil.

Eating cereals, with legumes or fruit, slows the digestive process, causing swelling or intestinal disorders.

Herbaceous Plants

I included in this category those foods that have similar characteristics to cereals, but do not really belong to that food family.

These include: quinoa, buckwheat, millet, amaranth, and sorghum, which can all be considered herbaceous plants.

As mentioned, they have characteristics comparable to cereals, even at the macro and micro nutrient level, but are more digestible as their grains are small, gluten-free, and without the outer coating.

The Healthy Natural Diet recommends their consumption in the same amount as cereals, mainly indicated for dinner, for their digestibility.

Legumes

Legumes are a natural food and definitely part of the Healthy Natural Diet.

They are quite difficult to digest because they contain starch, protein and fiber in abundance. As a consequence, it is advisable not to exceed in quantity, especially for those who are trying HND for the first time, as they may be accustomed to eating "traditional" and, most likely, have an unbalanced intestinal flora. Legumes are an important source of B Vitamins, Vitamin PP, folic acid and Vitamin H, as well as precious minerals such as iron, potassium and phosphorus.

We have already discussed most varieties of carbohydrates, proteins and fibers, as to be almost complete foods from the nutritional point of view, except for some anti-nutritional factors, generally of protein deprivation, which you can still inhibit almost completely with cooking.

The phasin for example, is a protein that causes problems to the small intestine, as well as trypsin inhibitors, which, from the very definition, inhibit the trypsin enzyme produced by the pancreas, responsible for the digestion of certain amino acids, especially arginine and lysine.

Some of these inhibitors are also heat-resistant, so are not completely inactivated by cooking.

Legumes also contain phytates, salts capable of joining to iron, calcium, zinc and phosphorus inhibiting its absorption.

The phytates are damaged but are not completely neutralized by cooking.

Germination is better than cooking as it guarantees a complete elimination of phytates, thus improving the digestive processes.

Lectin and saponine can also be found in legumes. These are anti-nutritional substances which facilitate the intestinal permeability, causing inflammation in the digestive system. These are also only partially eliminated by cooking.

To facilitate its cooking and the elimination of anti-nutritional factors, it has been suggested to soak legumes for several hours, taking care to eliminate the water and rinse before cooking.

Among the different types of legumes don't forget beans, chickpeas, soy, lupines, lentils, peas, and fava beans, all with many varieties among them: we may have green lentils, red, black and other types, as well as with other legumes.

Among the most digestible legumes are lentils and peas, which are the only ones that can be eaten raw, along with the fava beans.

In accordance with the Healthy Natural Diet, include legumes in your diet 4-5 times a week, in moderate amounts using the proper washing and cooking procedures.

After a certain period of HND, you can also combine cereals and legumes together, without other foods, except a good portion of raw vegetables before starting the meal.

An interesting way to consume legumes is to let them germinate, this way they become more digestible and with more nutritional properties.

Soybeans are also delicious to eat naturally, steamed in their pods.

It is important to know that all natural foods can be eaten easily, just by being mindful of the right way and the right amounts.

<u>Seeds</u>

Seeds are key nutrients in the Healthy Natural Diet, as they are rich in vitamins, minerals, complete protein, phytosterols, and fiber, but above all are the main source of essential and fundamental fatty acids, omega 6 and especially omega 3, precious natural anti-inflammatories.

They represent, along with avocado, the most natural seasoning. If you think that a seed can generate a plant, try to imagine how many precious properties are contained in these small granules.

Among the various choices on the market, don't forget flax seeds, hemp, Chia, very rich in omega 3, while sesame, sunflower, pumpkin, and poppy are excellent sources of omega 6.

In HND they are mainly used to prepare seasonings, but also salads, soups, purées, or other dishes prepared with cereals and vegetables by which they combine perfectly.

Seeds can be used safely even in fruit salads, to make them more tasty and complete from a nutritional point of view.

As natural fats, they guarantee a very high satiety because, thanks to chewing, we can make use of all those substances highly bioavailable and nutrients for our body.

Never miss seeds on your table and try to mix them and vary their consumption as much as possible.

As for quantity, 2-3 tablespoons per day are ideal for all possible benefits.

Oily Dried Fruit

Dried fruit, or fruit with shell, such as almonds, walnuts, hazelnuts, pecan nuts, macadamia nuts, pistachio nuts, cashew nuts and peanuts, have roughly the same properties as seeds, and also: good fats, good proteins, vitamins (E especially), fiber, important minerals such as iron and calcium.

In the Healthy Natural Diet it is recommended to use dried fruit as a condiment in salads or various dishes, as an alternative or in addition to traditional seeds.

However, It is important not to eat too much (this also applies to seeds), so as to not to create intestinal problems or excessive digestion times.

A handful of shelled fruit at lunch and dinner, is ideal to meet one's needs. Obviously, if associated with other fats such as seeds or avocados and olives, it is better to reduce consumption.

At times one can have a handful of dried fruit as a snack, in addition to fresh fruit, in particular after physical activity, which requires a greater caloric contribution.

Quality of seeds and dried fruits in general

You need to pay attention to quality, in particular on the origin of the product, as dried fruits or seeds from the United States, China or South East Asia often hide intensive farming and GMOs.

Also be careful when fruits are too smooth or too clean and without imperfections: the real dried fruits, such as classical country walnuts are small and ugly to look at, but certainly with a much higher nutritional potential and free from contamination. Also avoid packaged products, fried or baked and salty. Nutritional properties are lost during cooking, but mostly it's the fatty acids that are altered, becoming harmful for our body.

Quality is an important factor to consider, since on the market there are more unhealthy products, compared to those natural and free of contamination. Also, sometimes the price is a sign of quality: if there is a substantial difference there is a reason, in case of doubts inspect the product carefully.

Insights: Avocados, A Divine Gift

I've talked about different types of fat included in the Healthy Natural Diet, such as seeds, dried fruit, and olives, but also small quantities of good quality olive oil.

However, the element that best represents the HND thanks to its nutritional power is the avocado, which can also be used as a condiment and is probably the best food ever because it guarantees a degree of nourishment and satiation incomparable to other products.

To me, the avocado is the best of all fruits!

Unfortunately, it cannot be cultivated at all latitudes. But today, you can find this precious fruit even in new areas, for example, in Italy. In fact, Sicily and Calabria are good producers and their fruits are particularly tasty.

The avocado is eaten quite mature and to assess the degree of maturity, you should feel the softness.

There are some varieties of avocado, among which we remember the Haas, the Nabal, the Fuerte or Ettinger among the most popular and it is also possible to consume the seed, grating it in various preparations.

As for the properties, the avocado is rich in Vitamin E, Vitamin C, K and B group. It's a good source of fiber, antioxidants and precious carotenoids, as well as important minerals such as potassium, magnesium, calcium, iron, zinc and many others.

It is a precious source of omega-3, omega-6 and is useful in the prevention of many diseases, as well as in the detox process of the body or in skin and hair care.

You can have it regularly, without worrying about calories: there is no food on earth that, provided the same calories, can ensure such high nutritional power and satiety.

The Circadian Cycles

Before talking about the composition of meals to be distributed throughout the day, we need to consider the importance of circadian cycles or circadian rhythms.

The circadian cycles consist of a sort of internal clock, which regulates and synchronizes our body with the cycle of day and night, through natural stimuli such as sunlight or environmental temperature.

The circadian rhythms, through the endocrine system, are involved in various biological functions such as: sleep/wake stages, the parameters relating to body temperature and other apparatuses.

These phases are very important. In fact, people frequently subject to jet lag as well as night workers and shift workers may experience, sleep-related endocrine problems over time, but also gastrointestinal diseases.

There is therefore a strong bond between the introduction of food and the natural cycles to which the body is subject.

The HND method is fundamental to respect the circadian rhythms and reap the greatest benefits, as it is in harmony with nature.

The circadian cycles are 3 and last approximately 8 hours each.

The Morning Cycle or Eliminative Phase

This phase starts around 4 am and ends around noon. It can be defined as 'eliminative', since the body tends to clean up and eliminate toxins.

This also applies to excess water and fecal deposits, in fact, we tend to go to the bathroom more often during this period.

From a nutrition perspective , it is important to be in synergy with the purifying cycle.

It is therefore unnecessary, although often recommended, to eat hearty breakfasts by also combining different foods since it extends the digestive times and hinders the body functions involved.

A plentiful breakfast, rich in simple sugars and fat, like croissants for example, can cause fatigue and weight gain (due to the resulting insulin peak).

To avoid this, as a remedy, during the morning we resort to having several coffees.

Coffee is only an unhealthy palliative, and does not resolve the problem. Rather, it may accentuate it.

According to the HND method, during the eliminating cycle it is necessary to consume fresh aqueous fruit, rich in natural sugars.

This helps the purification of the body and, at the same time, introduces precious fuel, which allows a high performance in daily activities, with energy and clarity.

As for the eating methods, I always suggest the whole fruit and not extracts, juices or smoothies.

The whole fruit ensures a greater quantity of vitamins, antioxidants and a good fiber intake, keeping blood glucose levels constant. It favors the elimination of toxic substances from our body and satiety signals.

The Diurnal Cycle or Food Phase

The diurnal cycle or food phase includes the period in which it is necessary to eat and it includes both lunch and dinner.

It starts at noon and ends around 8 p.m. Therefore, it is appropriate to include meals within this timeframe.

According to the Healthy Natural Diet, lunch should be the most plentiful meal of the day.

A lunch allows you to have enough energy for the rest of the day and helps you avoid cravings throughout the afternoon.

The usual trend of recent times is to consume a late lunch on the go.

This leads to a hormonal imbalance to the circadian rhythms of our body: eating late often means altering satiety signals, creating the need for more frequent snacks and also delays the time of the dinner.

The consequences are a greater sense of fatigue, digestive problems and especially the difficulty in weight loss for those who want to lose weight.

To better deal with the food phase of the HND method, you would need to

- Have lunch from noon to 12.30 p.m.

- Have a snack around 4.30 p.m.

- Have dinner from 7.30 p.m. to 8pm at the latest.

As previously mentioned, lunch is the most important meal of the day in order to stay energized. Having a generous serving of whole grain cereals or tubers (potatoes, sweet potatoes, manioc or beets) and fresh seasonal vegetables is recommended.

Before all meals it is best to eat a portion of raw leafy green vegetables such as salads, spinach, chicory or radicchio with lemon juice, making sure to chew them very slowly.

Beginning the meal in this manner means increasing the absorption of nutrients (which takes place best in empty stomach conditions); it promotes digestion because of the many enzymes contained in raw vegetables, and slows glycemic peaks favouring the sense of satiety.

Even for a snack, my advice is to primarily eat seasonal fruits. If you have to face hard tasks, or when you feel very hungry, you can add a serving of dried nuts such as walnuts, almonds or pine nuts, natural, non-roasted and unsalted.

As a seasoning for lunch and dinner, HND essentially suggests the use of natural fats: olives, dried fruit and seeds of all types; when possible you can add some tasty slices of avocado rich in vitamins, antioxidants and high-quality fats.

Using these ingredients, you can create different dips which can make your dishes tasty and appetizing by just using natural foods.

Adding lemon juice is healthy because it increases the intake of Vitamin C and promotes the absorption of iron, as well as providing precious antioxidants. You can also consume small quantities of organic cold-pressed extra virgin olive oil.

The use of salt is not necessary and above all, it alters the true flavor of the foods. However, if necessary, I recommend using coarse salt, not washed and not mixed with other additives or substances, usually indicated on the labels.

The Night Cycle or Phase of the Immune System

It consists of the last 8 hours, from 8 p.m. to 4 a.m. and is the most important cycle since it does not strictly depend on our choices alone, but also on the hormonal and immune systems, which intervene with accurate self-regulating mechanisms.

These are important hours in which the self-healing mechanisms work hard to restore balance and detoxify the body.

It happens as in a fasting phase, which, upon awakening, is manifested with the typical eliminative effects of post-fasting, such as: rise in blood glucose, increase of cortisol, sometimes headaches, sore throat or joint aches and various weaknesses as the evidence of a cleaning activity in the body.

Obviously, the more the body is subject to unhealthy lifestyles, the greater the discomfort manifested in the morning, until the immune system will be able to restore its functions.

It is important to be mindful of this stage in order to get the best benefits the next day.

Late meals or snacks, drinking coffee or alcohol, and going to bed late at night, all hinder the cleansing process. These unruly behaviors are often the cause of morning fatigue. An excess of caffeinated beverages and/or simple sugar foods to cope with a state of lethargy do not solve the problem, but trigger a vicious circle with unforeseeable negative consequences of becoming increasingly tired and stressed.

Following the HND method doesn't mean to only eat properly, but to also adopt healthy habits and lifestyles. For example, going to bed early after digesting a light dinner will help facilitate the purifying and rebalancing that takes place during the night cycle.

The Combination of Foods

The Healthy Natural Diet consists of simple and nutritious meals.

You can create different combinations of foods, without neglecting their composition and circadian cycles, therefore, the distribution of meals throughout the day.

Exceptions may be made, especially in the initial phase of change, so that every person with different eating habits will have a personalized approach to this type of diet.

In general, to get the maximum benefit from the program, you need to follow some guidelines: during the eliminative phase, before noon, you have to help your body to implement the cleaning process.

All types of fruit are allowed; I suggest you start breakfast with fruits with a higher water content such as citrus fruits in general, melon, kiwi, berries or grapes.

By mid morning, in order to keep your blood sugar at constant levels, it's good to include an extra snack with fruit richer in calories such as bananas, pears, persimmons, and mangos. Also note that apples and pears are always recommended.

You can consume different fruits. The important thing is not mixing it with other foods to avoid obstructing and prolonging the digestive process, thus incurring in a fermentation process resulting in discomfort, abdominal swelling and interference in the assimilation of nutrients.

Fruit is a precious fuel, probably the best for the body as it has no waste and is especially available for energy purposes.

From noon to 8pm, we enter in the crucial assimilative phase.

Lunch, as previously stated, is the most important meal of the day because the body needs more energy to perform its functions effectively.

We are in the middle of the day, so it is essential to adequately feed the body but, at the same time, to not weigh it down with harmful foods that are not very compatible with our digestive system.

HND favours the consumption of whole grain cereals such as brown rice, barley, spelt, kamut or oats but also the herbaceous plants compared to cereals, including quinoa, buckwheat, millet or amaranth.

Herbaceous plants are good alternatives as they are gluten-free and therefore more digestible.

A good choice is made from tubers, especially potato or sweet potato, which is certainly the most natural variety with a higher content of vitamins and minerals and a starchy component more digestible and assimilable.

These foods are all rich in starch.

Before lunch we recommend a bowl of raw vegetables, preferably leafy greens rich in chlorophyll but also in vitamins, minerals, fiber and precious antioxidants.

You can quickly make unique, flavorful and satisfying dishes, without having to mix too many foods during the same meal.

In association with the cereals or starches there are the various types of vegetables.

There are no specific contraindications about it because you can consume all of these vegetables without problems.

Raw vegetables are healthier and richer in nutrients and enzymes that promote digestion.

It is not wrong to blanch vegetables, preferably in a special steamer with different pots, provided you always use very short cooking times (up to 5 minutes at most), in order to maintain a crunchy texture good not only for the taste, but also to avoid excessively altering their nutritional properties.

As for condiments, the use of natural fats in moderation is preferred, as they are healthier and more digestible.

Maximizing the amount of fat, such as adding large doses of oils means overly engaging the digestive system slowing down the assimilative processes to the point that it results in a feeling of tiredness and sleepiness right after the meal, which is preferable to avoid.

Olive, avocado and seed oils are the best solutions.

With these ingredients, it is also possible to prepare dips in order to make an even more tasty dish.

In the Healthy Natural Diet it is appropriate to introduce any type of spice such as: herbs, garlic, curry, turmeric, cumin, and chili (better if consumed fresh as to not excessively irritate the intestinal wall).

Playing with spices and seasonings in general contributes to the creation of diverse and tasty dishes. My advice is to continue experimenting with new and different preparations as you go.

For snacks, somewhere between lunch and dinner, it is recommended to have fresh fruit in order to keep blood sugar levels constant.

In the case of a stronger hunger or engaging in a sporting or other physically taxing activity, you can add a small portion of unsalted and non toasted dried fruit.

For dinner, the rules are basically the same as those of lunch, except for the main dish. For this course, the generous serving of whole grains will be significantly reduced and replaced at least 2-3 times per week with a predominantly protein rich food, such as legumes.

As for lunch, a good solution is the only dish.

Reducing the amount of food at dinner means encouraging the rapid absorption of nutrients in the assimilation phase, a prerequisite for an effective and complete night's rest.

Vegetable s are always a good choice, eaten hot in winter and cold in summer, made with all varieties of vegetables and with some tubers like potatoes, beets or squash to help thicken. You can add a handful of legumes, especially lentils or peas, among the most digestible, and whole pieces of vegetables, for added texture and crunch. Seeds or dried fruit will help give a more pleasant taste to the dish, while also providing those essential fatty acids necessary to satisfy the daily requirement.

Even the classic soups or "minestrone", mostly consumed in the winter, are excellent choices to add to the menu.

In this case small portions of whole grains, such as spelt or barley, can be added, without exceeding the consumption of legumes, less easy to digest.

With legumes, potatoes and the addition of spices, 1-2 times per week, you can make delicious meatballs or burgers to be cooked in the oven for a crispy and delicious texture.

Burgers and meatballs are not as filling as soups or minestrone and digestion is a bit more challenging. If consumed, however, with abundant portions of vegetables, the sense of satiety will improve dramatically.

With the use of tahini, which is a concentrate of omega 6 consisting of crushed sesame seeds, it is possible to prepare sauces or hummus of different types (with chickpeas or with aubergines for example), which can add great variety to your dinners. As a unique and nutritious addition to a dish I recommend a raw vegetable dip such as: celery, carrots, fennel, radicchio and salads.

Do not forget to add plenty fresh lemon juice, both in the preparations and as a seasoning for vegetables or salads.

Eating in a healthy way with a plant based diet is simple, nutritious and tasty. With a bit of imagination and following the basic principles of the Healthy Natural Diet you will experience a quick and healthy digestion, an optimal ideal weight and the right energy and vitality to face the most challenging activities in everyday life.

Summary

Daily example:

- BREAKFAST (eliminative phase): HND herbal tea, fresh seasonal fruit

- SNACK (eliminative phase): 1-2 seasonal fruits

- LUNCH (assimilative phase): 1 bowl of mixed salad (valerian, lettuce, radicchio), 1 dish of brown rice with seasonal vegetables

- SNACK (assimilative phase): fresh fruit salad with seeds and oily dried fruit.

- DINNER (assimilative phase): 1 dish of raw vegetables, vegetable purée with potatoes and lentils.

Preparation and Cooking Methods

In order to get the best benefits from food and assimilate vitamins, minerals and antioxidants in the most bioavailable and less invasive form for our body, it is necessary to eat mainly raw foods.

As early as in 1930, during the first World Congress of Microbiology held in Paris, Russian Dr. Kouchakoff had shown that eating cooked foods caused the body to enter into a leukocytosis process of increasing white blood cells, creating an inflammatory response similar to an external attack. [17]

The cooking process alters vitamins, such as Vitamin C and antioxidants, which are particularly sensitive to temperature increase.

One can easily experience that consuming a raw food, such as a fruit or a vegetable, provides a feeling of better digestibility compared to the same food consumed after cooking.

In the HND diet, there is a clear preference for raw foods.

In tropical countries or in areas where the sun shines for most of the year, there is an abundant variety of fruits and vegetables, juicy and full of nutrients, and so it is easier to eat raw foods.

For those who are trying the HND program for the first time, and are used to completely different eating methods, or for those who live in the Nordic countries and are not fortunate enough to have a variety of alternatives, eating raw is definitely more difficult and challenging because vegetables and fruits are usually imported in those countries; also, they are usually grown in greenhouses with aggressive methods and therefore have little flavor.

My advice in these cases is to gradually approach food changes without excessive stress on the timing.

To vary the diet or increase the number of possible combinations it may be necessary to include cooking alternatives at times.

Then, there are certain foods such as cereals or legumes that, in order to eliminate the anti-nutritional factors, must be cooked unless you opt for the sprouting process that requires a rather long period of time.

The general rule to adopt is 75% of the food to be raw and the rest cooked (in the summer season it can be up to 85-90%).

It is true that cooked food is not ideal, but eating 2/3 of raw food guarantees meeting the nutritional requirements for a good health and fitness.

If you have a tendency to prefer raw food or you live in climatic zones that permit this, increasing the percentage to 75-80 or even 90% is obviously advisable.

I mentioned cooked foods, but I also have to explain what I mean by cooking food and especially which methods can be used in the Healthy Natural Diet.

For cereals and legumes, cooking in boiling water is required. For the rest, thus essential for vegetables, the only possible alternative to raw is steaming.

It is preferable to use a steamer with two baskets. The first, in contact with the heat contains boiling water. The second basket contains vegetables which cook thanks to the steam below. To preserve as much as possible vitamins and antioxidants, cooking time must be quite rapid (within 5 minutes), to also preserve food texture.

The remaining water can be used as a broth or as a kind of herbal tea, or simply for watering flowers and plants for a greater nourishment.

Even cooking in a pressure cooker is recommended, but only for cereals and legumes to reduce cooking times. However, for vegetables, it appears to be an "aggressive" approach.

Other methods of cooking vegetables are not recommended; however zucchini and peppers can be stuffed with the skin or in the oven.

This is acceptable because as already said, it is not essential that 100% of the diet consists of only raw foods.

In this case the baking process may alter vitamins and phytochemicals as they are particularly sensitive, but if done properly, and without burning the food, it does not appear to be harmful.

As for potatoes and tubers, oven cooking is a good alternative to boiling.

Fry and grill, however, are not permitted in HND.

Grilled or roasted vegetables lose much of their nutritional value and can also become harmful due to the charring on the surface.

However, as in any other field, there are often exceptions, while it is important The important to stick to the rules and procedures as much as possible.

Insights: Microwave Cooking

To speed up the process of heating food, especially in local and fast food centers, a microwave oven is often being used.

The food cooking in the microwave is heated by the interaction of the food with electromagnetic fields emitted in the microwave spectrum. In a conventional oven, electric or gas heat is transmitted by radiation and by conduction, in a direction that comes from the outer layers to the innermost ones. Instead, when using the microwave it is possible that the central part of the food, especially if contains water or lipids, warms up much faster than the outside. In this case food heated in the microwave could have the disadvantage of an uneven distribution of heat.

As a first consequence, it experiences loss and degradation, especially in vitamins or antioxidants that are particularly sensitive to heat, as well as denaturation and rancidity processes related to fat and protein.

The introduction into the human body of molecules and energies to which it is not used to is likely to have adverse effects more than positive: the microwaves produced by alternating currents, in fact, lead millions of polarity reversals per second in each molecule of food that it strikes. Production of unnatural molecules is inevitable.

Some research has shown a correlation between microwave cooking and possible carcinogenic effects. [18]

You should also pay attention to plastic containers which are commonly used to heat food in the microwave because they can cause the release of bisphenol A, a known endocrine disruptor.

Summary

Methods of Preparation And Cooking Of Food In Hnd

- *70% raw, 30% cooked*

- *Recommended cooking: steam in a special steamer or pressure cooker*

- *Acceptable cooking: the oven (no microwave)*

- *Cooking methods not permitted: grill, barbecue, fry*

Quantity and Distribution of Food in the Day

To apply the Healthy Natural Diet, you must have an initial consultation, which includes the state of health, the habits and the lifestyle of the subject.

It is advisable to continue with indirect calorimetry (or use different mathematical equations, scientifically validated) in order to evaluate caloric expenditure, useful to better define the amount of food to be introduced in every meal.

These evaluations must be performed by someone who is professionally qualified to do so and, able to detect and manage, if necessary any problems that may arise.

Not everyone starts from the same conditions and with the same habits.

You need to consider: age, work, family commitments and the lifestyle of each individual.

It is true that there are rules that can apply to everyone, but it is also true that certain categories of people, such as shift workers or athletes involved in important competitions, are subject to unique daily routines and unorthodox schedules that may require special adjustments to fit their respective needs. Generally, the day is divided into 5 meals. This is the best strategy: breakfast, lunch, dinner and two snacks mid-morning and mid-afternoon.

The division into 5 meals allows one to maintain blood glucose in constant levels, avoiding losses or significant blood glucose elevations.

The amount is not a fundamental and indispensable factor because, as already explained, eating healthy and natural foods leads the body to quickly recognize the signals of satiety.

Around The Water

Today, it is generally accepted, both in the academic environment and in public opinion, that drinking plenty of water is good for you and helps maintaining a good state of health.

I do not fully agree with this theory because, as evidence shows, there is a substantial difference between the water inside our cells and the water we drink.

It is important to understand how our body works and why drinking a lot is actually unnecessary.

Water in our body is mostly contained in our lean mass (hence, all non-fat tissue), metabolically active in carrying out the main functions.

Conversely, the fat mass is anhydrous (devoid of water) and its function is to store energy.

This is why thin individuals need to drink more whereas overweight and morbidly obese people drink a lot less, as they have a lower percentage of lean mass.

To better explain this concept: human beings 'typically' have body water percentages of around 65-70%, whereas in those that are overweight, it can be even less than 50%!

Water requirements in those individuals are definitely lower, in fact, in average, their thirst stimulus is far less frequent.

Water, Water Retention And Health

It often happens that overweight people or others with a fat-mass above average are recommended to drink more water for several reasons such as: improvement of overall health, renal function, toning, skin protection, preventing water retention, etc.

These are certainly all important aspects to be taken into consideration; however, to drink more water without changing our lifestyle, improving our diet and increasing our physical activity would not help resolve those persisting issues and would not result in significant improvements in our overall appearance. Whereas, a radical change in our routine by approaching our HND program, would certainly lead to results far more effective and remarkable.

The reason for this is fairly simple: by drinking more water I will neither build more lean mass and eliminate fat, nor will I increase the blood perfusion and enhance the microcirculation.

In order to achieve tangible benefits you need to change your lifestyle, avoiding physical inactivity as well as an improper, non-natural diet.

Water Retention

Water retention, often confused by other names and with other matters, is nothing but water imbalance, meaning that a higher percentage of liquids within the intercellular spaces are accumulated excessively causing swellings and edemas especially in joint areas.

Water retention can be very dangerous for our overall health when derived from renal insufficiency or kidney diseases in general: from a nutritional perspective, this issues are the result of an unhealthy lifestyle, which, if untreated, can worsen alarmingly.

This disease affects especially overweight, sedentary people, following an unhealthy diet, rich in fats, proteins and processed foods incompatible with our digestive system.

In these circumstances waste products accumulate in the interstitial spaces where they remain persistently due to the poor microcirculation inhibited by the excessive fat mass.

These fat masses are aggravated by the lack of physical activity which contributes to further reduce the microcirculation, crucial in supplying cells with nutrients and removing waste products derived from all metabolic and digestive processes. This can be very harmful to our health.

In fact, waste products, also called toxins, if not properly eliminated from our vascular and lymphatic system, may cause inflammatory processes that can eventually lead to severe pathologies.

It is important to remember that the baselines of all diseases are always inflammatory processes; therefore, minimizing inflammation helps you keep good health in the long term.

Water retention is among the main causes of inflammation linked to lifestyle, healthy/unhealthy eating and physical activity/inactivity.

Different Water

Before introducing the topic related to bottled water, it is important to remember that the water we commonly drink is totally different from the water present in our cells and, as can be seen later, not exactly healthy.

The best water that provides essential, bio-available micronutrients to our body is the one contained in plant-based foods, especially fruit and vegetable. This is devoid of contamination and it's what the HND model supports.

Requirements

When following the HND program, one's daily water supply is almost totally provided by fruits and vegetables; However, it is important to not neglect thirst stimulus that can be more frequent in the summer or during and right after a workout session, especially when carried out indoors or with an excess of heat and humidity. In fact, in these circumstances, the dehydration is considerably higher.

Another important rule, according to the HND program, is to drink as little as possible during mealtimes (given that meals are already rich in vegetable portions), in order to avoid "diluting" digestive enzymes and cause bad digestion.

Water And Physical Activity

During workouts and sporting events, water intake becomes necessary to guarantee a good performance and from a health perspective, first and foremost, so much so that an excessive dehydration can cause heat-stroke and even death.

Therefore, in these circumstances, especially with high heat and humidity, drinking water or other liquids is fundamental.

I often advise athletes that by eating small amounts of fruit on an ongoing basis during sporting activities, one can largely meet the requirements of liquids and avoid dehydration, also achieving significant improvements in terms of performance.

In fact, fruit contains very important nutrients such as: sugars, vitamins, minerals and antioxidants that makes it unnecessary to consume industrial supplements as the latter do not offer the same benefits and do not have the same bio-availability as natural foods.

In conclusion:

Water is an essential element for our body but it is extremely important to consider which form we are taking in.

Bottled Waters

Following this introduction on the topic related to water, let us now analyze what's behind the "world" of bottled waters available in supermarkets, restaurants and retail industry in general.

First, there is a big difference between bottled water and drinkable water and it's just not true that bottled water is healthier and safer, so much so that mineral waters, considered as "therapeutic" may contain arsenic, cadmium, aluminium, barium, etc., which are much lower and often not admitted in drinkable water (check the table below); moreover, as for the arsenic, producers do not have the obligation to highlight its levels on the label.

It is also important to note that water collection and bottling processes may take place miles away from the source and that several days or weeks may pass from the collection to the final consumer which certainly results in a lower quality although the product is well marketed and advertised in such a way to mislead buyers.

In addition, it is useful to consider that 80% of water is sold in PET bottles in which bisphenol A is used. This is an extremely harmful substance, responsible for a large number of severe pathologies including prostatic cancer, problems during pregnancy, and also affecting the fetus.

Limit Value of substances contained in drinkable and bottled water		
	Limit Value **drinkable water** Decree Law. 31/2001	Limit Value **bottled water** Decree 542/92 – MD 31/05/2001
Arsenic-total($\mu g/l$)	10	50
Barium ($\mu g/l$)	-	1
Chromium ($\mu g/l$)	50	50
Lead ($\mu g/l$)	10-25	10

Nitrates (mg/l)	50	45-10*
Aluminium (μg/l)	200	No limit
Iron (μg/l)	200	No limit
Manganese (μg/l)	50	2000
Fluoride (mg/l)	1,50	No limit

Tap Water

Tap water is much safer due to the greater attention it is subjected to regarding the substances value limits and the micro-bacteriological controls. However, it cannot be compared to cellular water since there are no disinfection systems, chlorination in particular, that would make tap water as pure as the cellular water.

In addition, plumbing systems can be several kilometers in length, depriving water of its taste-olfactory properties and making it undrinkable, hence replaceable by mineral waters.

Pipelines represent a limitation not just regarding the organoleptic aspect but, very likely also with reference to pollutants coming from the soil.

In fact, the ground collects various residues from the environment, in particular from rain, factory farming and intensive livestock breeding.

These extremely dangerous substances are hardly eliminated completely by wastewater treatment systems and may enter into the water supply network.

In conclusion:

All these considerations are not intended to scare but simply to highlight the importance to pay close attention when choosing which water to drink, as sometimes the indications we are given are somehow inaccurate.

Ultimately, according to the HND model, the best water at our disposal is the one contained in seasonal fruits and vegetables, of course, being vigilant as to their quality as well.

Drinking During Meals

Drinking a lot is not essential for the wellness of the individual because the best bio-available water is contained in fruits and vegetables.

My advice is to drink when thirsty and, if possible, to avoid doing it during meals. Introducing liquids while eating ends up excessively diluting the precious digestive enzymes used in food break down.

This may result in digestive time delays with the addition of the fermentation process, which contributes to creating a sense of fullness and abdominal swelling that one may often feel after meals.

HND eating is rather simple and totally plant-based, consequently rich with water based foods.

The stimulus of thirst following this type of eating, is felt less. If however you need to drink, it is best done 15-20 minutes before a meal or during,but in small sips.

Insights: Juices and Smoothies

It is common practice in recent times resort to various juices and smoothies, consumed both in the home and in public places.

If we must choose between a coffee or a juice, the second option is definitely healthier, but from my point of view excess consumption of these juices does not guarantee specific benefits to the body; in some occasions, it may even be counterproductive, because the excessive concentration of sugars which, although of excellent origin, are not adequately regulated by the fiber and other compounds present in the whole fruit.

This implies an increase in the blood sugar spike and insulin production with consequent effects caused by rebound hypoglycemia. Remember, the nutritional power of a whole fruit is definitely higher than the same fruit shakes or juices, so much so that eating fruits, for example 2-3 less, gives a sense of satiety even more relevant than 5-6 fruits shakes or juices, which have a much lower satiating power.

This is not only due to the loss of fiber, vitamins or various phytochemicals, which degrade with the processing, but, more importantly, by the absence of chewing, an important process in triggering a series of physiological mechanisms aimed at achieving satiety.

The following examines the differences between smoothies and juices.

The smoothie is probably the healthiest option, since the fiber is not eliminated, so it is present in the preparation although perhaps unwelcome to delicate palates. The fiber is present, but separated from the juice, and so does not present the same advantages and the same properties of the fruit consumed whole.

Smoothies and juices, from my point of view, do not have big differences: the juices have a slower rate of squeezing, and also don't contain steel blades, as does the smoothie, but an auger aimed at protecting the sensitive vitamins and antioxidants to oxidation due on metal.

In the first, there is probably something better, but is more a marketing strategy than a real benefit to the body.

A good compromise is represented by the pressing of the food, even if when you go to edit a fruit or a vegetable, the important and sensitive nutrients decrease significantly.

The best indication, according to the HND method, is always to eat the whole food.

We must respect the limits imposed by nature and our physiology, after all, if we have the teeth there is a reason!

As mentioned before, at the bar, in the breaks or during the aperitif it is preferable to drink a juice or smoothie made of fruits and/or vegetables than a coffee, chocolate or even worse, an alcoholic beverage but this does not justify an abundant use in everyday life.

For sports, these drinks may be useful both during the performance, may be diluted in water, and also in the very important post recovery activities, in order to promptly recharge the glycogen stores and various minerals, when due to adrenaline or other endorphins present after physical exertion, the sense of hunger remains partially inhibited.

Omega 3, Vitamin B12 And Iron

It is commonly believed that vegetable diets are lacking some essential nutrients. To disprove this thought, here are some insights on some of the most frequently discussed.

Omega 3

The precursor of reference is the alpha linolenic acid, from which derive the various families including EPA and DHA.

Emphasizing: Alpha linolenic acid is considered the essential fat because this is what the others are derived from.

It is therefore not necessary to address EPA and DHA separately, because these are no more than derivatives of essential fatty acid reference (alpha linolenic precisely).

The alpha-linolenic acid (ALA), once introduced into our body through eating, is metabolized and converted into EPA and DHA.

There would be as explained by various researchers a "conversion efficiency". [19]

The body can produce omega-3 long chain fatty acid from its natural precursor, alpha-linolenic acid, which is the only omega-3 essential fatty acid, which is derived mainly from plant sources (seed flax, hemp or Chia, walnuts, soy, etc.).

Benefits Of Omega 3

Let's examine the utility of omega 3 in our body.

According to various scientific sources [16,19,20,21,22,23,24,25,26] these fats are extremely important because:

- They reduce blood triglycerides up to 40%.

- They lead to a reduction in blood pressure.

- They have effects on memory, concentration and learning.

- They are essential because the skin remains healthy and vital and combats aging.

- They hinder the formation of thrombi, reducing the risk of heart attack.

- They decrease the symptoms of angina and heart palpitations.

- They are essential in gestation

- They reduce the risk of macular degeneration of the eyes

- They improve mood and forms of depression.

- They strengthen the immune system

- They improve symptoms of Alzheimer's, Crohn's disease, Lupus, Schizophrenia, bipolar disorders, premenstrual syndrome and painful menstruation.

Sources Of Omega 3: The Hoax Of Fish

It is necessary to clarify the sources of Omega 3 because there is always some confusion due to the economic interests of the fish market.

Let's examine the following table which compares plant and animal sources (fish only) of omega 3.

OMEGA 3 SOURCES (g/100g of product)

ANIMAL DERIVATION	PLANT DERIVATION
Fresh sardines 1.73	Linseed oil 66
Eel 1.30	Flax seeds 32
Fresh herring 1.09	Hemp oil 18
Fresh salmon 0.89	Walnut oil 14
Fresh tuna 0.80	Cooked soy 11
Mackerel 0.73	Soy oil 7.6
Fresh sea bass 0.48	Walnut 6.5
Fresh sea bream 0.46	Wheat germ 5.4
	Pumpkin seeds 5

Vegetables, as well as having higher amounts of omega-3, compared to those of animal origin, also have a greater variety of choice: oils, seeds, nuts, some vegetables and vegetable drinks.

A recent medical and scientific research conducted on over 19,000 people in the United Kingdom (2010), the results of which have been made public in an article recently published in the American Journal of Clinical Nutrition, notes that the intake of omega 3 is more efficient when derived from plants. [19]

It should also noted that taking omega 3 cannot be assured when eating fish.

To avoid contamination of a different nature, and to be consumed safely, the fish must be cooked. As a result, the rather high temperatures, when cooked for some time, cause an alteration in the structure of the fat.

The omega 3, in fact, is a particularly sensitive fat (because of the double bonds of the carbon atoms), turns out to be unstable to heat. [27,28]

Imagine what can happen when cooked to 200 degrees over time!

The fat is denatured, that completely changes its structure, undergoing rancidity processes and becoming a saturated fat.

The studies done with the reduction of inflammation and cardiovascular problems, for the most part, considered the Eskimo population and referred to a consumption of fish of excellent quality, certainly not bred, therefore free and in clean seas.

But above all, and I want to emphasize, it is referred to the animal's power mode, which was mainly raw.

Compared to that time, many things have changed, especially the pollution of the seas and the methods of supplying fish (today, most are farmed).

It should also be added that from the discarded fish you get various oils that are encapsulated and sold as omega 3 supplements with high economic benefits.

Vitamin B12

Vitamin B12 or cyanocobalamin, has been the subject of many debates concerning plant nutrition because it is a common idea that those who follow a diet without animal proteins face deficiencies, in particular that of Vitamin B12.

Many vegans are convinced of this because, while proteins, omega 3 fatty acids, and other trace elements can now be taken in larger quantities, in the plant kingdom, this is not true for Vitamin B12, which adds to the confusion.

Vitamin B12 is not "naturally" contained in any food as it is a molecule produced by bacteria, mushrooms and algae. [16,19,26].

It is therefore incorrect to think that it is present in meat or any other product of animal origin: the animal, in fact, contains Vitamin B12 only because it is fed with food containing an artificial supplement of B12, or simply takes it from the soil present in the plants they eat. [19,26].

Deficiency of B12, in human beings (I refer to all human beings and not only to vegans), is largely due to a condition of malabsorption (therefore not lack of assumption), due to several factors: problems related to the intestinal flora (dysbiosis), cobalt deficiency, enzymatic factors; bad eating habits (excess of simple sugars, lactose and milk caseins, proteins, as well as white flours and industrial gluten), prolonged and frequent use of antacids, antibiotics, antidepressants, NSAIDs and other drugs; alteration of the intrinsic factor (a glycoprotein present in the gastric juice), cases of gastric resections, tumors or surgical interventions affecting the stomach or intestine (in particular the section called Ileo, where the Vitamin is absorbed), celiac disease or Crohn's disease; old age: as you get older you may not be able to assimilate cobalamin properly because of the lack of hydrochloric acid in your stomach.

Even the habits of unhealthy lifestyles, such as excessive smoking and alcohol negatively affect the absorption of B12.

Where to Take Vitamin B12

According to some studies [19,29,30,31], small amounts of Vitamin B12, used to meet the daily requirement, (2-4 micrograms), are present in the skin or on the exterior of some vegetables especially if they are grown in soils that take non-invasive methods, therefore, with a high presence of bacteria.

Our daily diet should include cobalt-rich foods, and of course, the HND system provides them in abundance: radicchio, beets, cabbage, tomatoes, lettuce, onions; fruits such as apples, pears, apricots, cherries, figs, plums, etc. and even vegetables, especially beans and lentils. [19,26,32,33]

Even algae is an excellent source of B12, but unfortunately the marine waters are not the healthiest, so basically the HND system does not recommend consumption, except rarely and in small quantities. There is an algae (actually not a real algae), the Klamath, that does not come from the sea, but from a pristine lake, which may allow a higher consumption. [33]

We must add that a fraction of B12 can be reabsorbed in the enterohepatic circulation, so, you can also use this function.

To reiterate, in the vast majority of cases, lack of B12 is exclusively due to an absorption problem!

Taking supplements, therefore, is not necessary, because the extract of a particular substance, especially if made chemically, does not have the same bioavailability as those derived from living foods (fruits and vegetables, mostly raw and cultivated without the use of pesticides and contaminants).

The amount of Vitamin B12, enough to cover our needs, is minimal and the HND diet amply provides coverage, including cobalt, necessary for its formation.

As mentioned above, almost all the problems are related to malabsorption, essentially due to incorrect habits: switch to a natural diet, and then follow the HND method, which in addition to nutrition is adaptable to most lifestyles, may make improvements and restore the gastrointestinal mucous membranes, as well as rebalance the bacterial flora in such a way as to ensure an adequate absorption of Vitamin B12.

Iron

Iron (Fe), is a transition metal, an important mineral as the cofactor of numerous proteins belonging to three main classes: the heme proteins, such as hemoglobin or myoglobin, Fe-sulfur proteins (with iron bound to cysteines), and the proteins bound to the iron transport, such as transparencies. [16]

It plays an essential role in the transport and utilization of oxygen and for the operation of various enzymes.

There are two main forms of iron: heme Fe, coming from foods of animal origin and non-heme Fe, present in foods of plant origin. [16,19]

Requirements vary by age and gender, but also depend a lot on losses, especially for women during the menstrual cycle, but also in the urine, faeces or sweat.

People most at risk are women of childbearing age, pregnant and more (for the growth of the placenta, needs of the fetus, or the increased blood volume during pregnancy), and also children during growth stages or endurance/ultra-endurance athletes. [16]

It is important to dispel the myth that when experiencing an iron deficiency, you must consume meat, especially red meat.

From personal experience, I have seen people with ferritin below recommended exposure limits, consume more than 3-4 times per week of red meat cooked rare, without finding any improvement.

In my opinion there are more dangerous consequences derived by the high consumption of red meat, whereas low levels of iron, iron deficiency, is almost always caused by conditions of malabsorption due to improper eating habits and lifestyles.

The iron is assimilated in an acid environment in which a reduction of hydrochloric acid in the stomach, common in the elderly or those who make frequent use of antacids, may hinder absorption.

The excess of free radicals too, due to unhealthy lifestyles, consumption of alcohol, smoking or drugs, help to inhibit the absorption of this mineral. [16,19]

Much the same happens in those that eat "bad" foods, which consequently promote the increase of free radicals and lack Vitamin C.

It is the case of meat and animal protein in general that sometimes, especially if consumed in excess, leads to inflammation and minor bleeding in the digestive tract.

Even the industrial sugar, contained in sweets, candy, baked goods or fizzy drinks, do not seem to promote iron absorption as phytates, the content in some vegetables (such as spinach or beets), in some legumes, cereals or seeds. [19,34,35,36].

Coffee and all caffeinated substances also inhibit the absorption of iron. [19,37,38]

HND and Iron

The problem of iron deficiency is clearly tied to unhealthy habits that inhibit its absorption, as well as certain stages of life, such as growth or pregnancy, which require significant increases.

Women, because of their menstrual cycle, have an increased need, as do athletes (running, especially if prolonged over time, leads to haemolysis of red blood cells resulting in the loss of iron).

Focusing only on the intake of the mineral means losing sight of the problem: you can introduce iron in abundance, but if it is not assimilated, or is lost, you need to raise the dosage.

The Healthy Natural Diet is a lifestyle system that covers only natural, non inflammatory foods.

Those who follow the Healthy Natural Diet, usually avoid pro-inflammatory foods, as well as unhealthy habits such as smoking, drug and alcohol use.

Industrial sugar and white flour, void of nutrients, are replaced by fruit sugars and whole grains that not only provide important vitamins and antioxidants, but are also an excellent source of iron.

HND does not include the consumption of coffee or other Nerve Substances. They are rich in biologically active trace elements, such as Vitamin C, which promote good iron absorption. [16,19]

Having clarified that the problem of iron deficiency is not only related to its introduction, you must remember that the plant kingdom, is a far greater source than the animal: legumes, nuts, seeds, but also whole grains, and especially vegetables, food cornerstones of the Healthy Natural Diet, are rich in iron. [16,19,39,40].

My advice is to add fresh squeezed lemon juice, providing good quantities of Vitamin C, to ensure that the non-haem iron absorption (so of vegetable origin) is complete.

The resort integration is not advisable because, not only does it not correct the bad habits, which are the true cause of the problem, but is also likely to introduce an excess of the mineral, with possible damage to the body.

Exceptions without Consequences to the HND Method

A question that many people ask me is the following: "If I go out to eat, or to have dinner on the weekend, or at a friend's house, or with relatives or various events, how should I behave?"

My answer is: "Do what your new awareness suggests to you".

What does this phrase mean?

It is normal for a person at the beginning of a change, pledging to improve their lifestyle, may not be fully aware of their behaviours.

While sharing the HND program, it is not easy to have ideas, flexibility and familiarity in implementing this particular diet.

From my point of view, awareness can only be achieved after having experienced and consolidated it; but if you are convinced of its value, in a short time, it will lead you to change your way of thinking, and to operate and manage the various food choices more easily.

Keeping an open mind and being willing to learn are the necessary conditions to improve both the lifestyle and the state of psycho-physical well being.

Returning to the initial discussion, we must not be afraid to go out and eat something that the HND diet does not support.

How can a meal affect the approximately 30/35 meals (including snacks) of the week?

Diet cannot be an imposition, but a choice that you want to make: "I eat this way because I want to and it makes me feel good!"

With the formation of new habits, you will automatically avoid consuming certain foods and even outside the home, you will know how to compensate in the most appropriate way.

Follow a Single Line and Not Millions of People

It is one of the many mistakes that are often committed. Many people ask me: "I do not know what path to follow, I have two different voices in my head..." I answer them, "You do not have two voices, it is probably a crowd!"

Now that the issue of nutrition has become so important and so popular, control over nutrition has been lost as a science monitored by professionals and increasingly manipulated by people without any university qualifications.

The causes of this confusion are manifold.

Of course, there is also the involvement of a health system that needs to be reviewed, and which has contributed to the success of various professional figures, that are no longer up to date.

Medical training prefers to focus on "drug treatment" as the solution to various physical and emotional problems, rather than focusing on the preventive power of food and taking the actions needed to achieve health and well-being. The word "diet" is now only understood as a purely medical concept and should be extended to that of an idea of well-being, harmony and physical fitness.

To this, a ruthless marketing industry was added, selling a massive variety of products and supplements, which created confusion in consumers.

We need to clarify and understand how to behave.

We are also bombarded by opposing views coming from a variety of sources: television, radio, street advertising, friends, clubs, gyms, personal trainers, nutritionists and doctors: they all claim different paths. At this point the question arises: "Who do I listen to? Who do I trust? "My advice is to take a single path and give yourself time to understand it thoroughly.

Only results count, but action is needed: without action, nothing is achieved!

Some people, especially in the summer, follow different paths, with the intention of losing weight, but with discouraging results; because there was no awareness about it, but just a thought dictated by instinct to want to lose weight and want to do it quickly.

As I've said, the goal should not be aimed at weight loss, but at the change in habits, then lifestyle. Weight loss will then be a side effect of making healthier choices one day to the next. As the HND method proposes, only in this way can lasting results be achieved.

Give the HND program a try and give yourself the time to experience the results. You will not look back. You will reach your desired goals!

HND LIFESTYLE

The HND method is also a guide to a better management of your day, trying to follow a healthy lifestyle in harmony with the nature around us.

Eating healthy is not sufficient to determine our quality of life.

In this chapter we propose an example of how you can organize your day in order to get the maximum benefit from the Healthy Natural Diet.

Obviously, these are general instructions. However, it is known that certain jobs or important commitments can slow down the success of the program, but this can be overcome by modifying some small habits.

Importance of Sleep and Morning Routines

Waking up in the morning, having slept enough, is healthy and regenerating for the body.

The amount of sleep is not important, but the quality: going to bed early at approximately 9.30 p.m. in the winter and around 10.30 p.m. in the summer, is ideal for a deep and rejuvenating sleep.

Even 5-6 hours of sleep, without awakening, are much more effective than more hours at different times of the circadian cycles.

Sleep respecting these simple rules also means having the benefit of body weight reduction.

As soon as you wake up, you should expose yourself to the morning air and take a dozen deep breaths, using the contraction of the diaphragm, to collect as much air as possible.

Then you should, especially during the summer or when the sun is shining, get some sun for 15 to 30 minutes (even more if you get a chance). All the while staying mindful of your breathing, possibly in meditation. This will also give you a good dose of Vitamin D which is essential for optimal functioning of the immune system. At the beginning of the day, before breakfast, it's important to move your body, followed by a phase of stretching. These exercises help to extend the spine, warm up the joints, and relax various muscle groups of the body.

We are aware that not everyone has the time to carry out such a morning routine.

On the other hand, aches and pains, various problems and also a high rate of stress, are partly due to a negligence of moving one's body for an extended time.

In the beginning, adopting these good habits can be tiring, because they require a level of organization, but over time, the payoff of good health is well worth the effort. Getting up and feeling good with a good dose of energy and vitality means facing the day in a more productive and effective way.

Insights: HND Infusion

Being in the habit of drinking coffee as soon as you wake up, means causing an excess of acidity and consequent irritability of the gastric and intestinal mucous membranes. This is not really healthy for your body, as it is coming off of the elminative cycle and cleansing phase. And for those that are sensitive, they will notice a sense of acidity, reflux, or annoyance caused by the consumption of coffee or caffeinated substances in general (tea or cocoa for example).

Worse still, cappuccino, in which there is a combination of milk and coffee, produces tannate of albumin, a substance that is metabolized for more than 3 hours. The whey caseins, moreover, form a sort of sticky mucus that settles on the intestinal walls, hindering the processes of absorption of nutrients and causing inflammatory reactions.

Often, it is precisely these established habits that cause the problems that are most difficult to treat.

Go ahead and drink something, as long as it is not harmful!

It is well known that after water, tea, but above all coffee, are among the most consumed drinks on earth, not only for their taste, but also their use in social situations and rituals.

Healthy alternatives are possible. In the Healthy Natural Diet, I recommend an infused beverage of some kind that can be changed according to personal tastes and preferences.

There are many different flavors and compositions available on the market.

A good suggestion is to make yourself an infusion, decoction or maceration, choosing the herbs carefully, according to your preferences and desired properties: anti-inflammatory and expectorant like linden, elderberry, sage, mint, Echinacea; energetic with ginseng, Guarana, Ginkgo or royal jelly; detoxifying herbs such as thistle, artichoke, red currants.

HND Infusion

For a classic herbal tea, before pouring water into the glass or the cup, we add:

- A pinch of unwashed and unrefined integral salt

- 2-3 slices of fresh ginger

- The juice of one lemon (after adding water), when the preparation is warm and drinkable.

Integral salt, uncooked and natural, is rich in precious minerals that, especially after a good night rest, when liquids and mineral salts are removed via breath and perspiration, helps to restore these precious substances.

It is also suitable for hypertension, because the problem of high blood pressure is predominantly related to the highly toxic and pro-inflammatory foods eaten in an unhealthy lifestyle. A pinch of integral salt is not a problem, especially if you follow the HND protocol rich in fruits and vegetables. Ginger is a powerful natural anti-inflammatory, analgesic, painkiller, and of great benefit to the immune system.

It helps regulate the gastrointestinal system, and it is advisable to take even small pieces after meals to aid digestion. It is important to consume the ginger fresh and raw if possible, chew it as well after drinking the tea.

The benefits of lemons are universally understood, lemons are high in Vitamin C as well as minerals and antioxidants; it is great for the immune system and maintains the body's pH balance.

It has excellent cleansing properties, antibiotic and preventative functions against many diseases.

It helps the absorption of iron and other minerals.

The herbs contained in the infusion/herbal tea, combined with the valuable properties of these elements, is of great help and benefit, especially in the morning, in the purifying phase, but also during the day, replacing classic coffee, unhealthy for the body.

As for the seasons, in cold periods, it is preferable to consume a hot drink. In the morning, however, there are those who prefer to drink a lukewarm herbal tea; if you want to have something fresh, you can put the preparation in the refrigerator the night before and drink it the next morning, taking care to add the lemon juice, squeezed at that time, to avoid loss of nutrients.

Insights: Coffee and Caffeinated Substances

Coffee, as well as caffeinated beverages in general, such as tea or cocoa, and dairy products are not healthy for our body.

The caffeinated foods are a particular group of foods or drinks that contain natural alkaloids such as caffeine or derivatives (such as theophylline or theobromine, contained in cocoa and tea, respectively). You can add to this family all those soft drinks based on cola or other energy drinks, commercially available, high in xanthine.

I would like to focus mainly on coffee, tea, and cocoa, which often result in conflicted opinions.

The Healthy Natural Diet does not recommend consumption of these drinks in everyday life, because caffeine has the ability to irritate the gastrointestinal mucosa. [64,65]

An excessive consumption can lead to serious problems such as reflux and gastritis, up to gastric ulcers, especially if combined with other bad habits, such as smoking or alcohol. [19]

In the most sensitive subjects it may also cause anxiety, nervousness, irritability and insomnia up to arrhythmias and heart palpitations. [20,21,22,23]

Behind coffee consumption and caffeinated drinks in general, there is a massively profitable industry promoting the consumption of these beverages so it is highly unlikely that they would highlight any negative effects to the body; many have even gone so far as to support the exact opposite!

Correlations between certain types of cancers have emerged, such as the ovaries, bladder, stomach, pancreas, and intestines cancer, that may be related to excessive consumption of coffee. [24,25,26]

This is attributed to the presence of polycyclic aromatic hydrocarbons (PAH), which are only some of the different chemicals detected.

The oxalic acid, present in the drink, inhibits the absorption of calcium: the tannins, that of iron and Vitamin C, especially when eaten close to a meal.

In addition to digestive problems, also due to its laxative effect, coffee also affects the renal system, as a single cup takes up to 20 hours to finally be metabolized because of the many acidic substances contained therein.

Finally, it is important to remember, the problems linked to the alteration of sleep, which can occur even with having a single cup, consumed in the morning. [27,28]

These problems also end up altering the circadian cycles, vital in safeguarding our health and well-being.

It's a bit of an unhealthy habit the one concerning coffee consumption: almost all drink it, especially in the morning, because, due to the eliminative cycle, leading to eliminate various toxins in the body, we often feel tired and exhausted due to an unhealthy lifestyle and especially if it also includes junk foods.

The use of coffee to improve one's mood is still at best a short-lived solution because after the effects of the adrenaline stimulation wear off, there is a subsequent fatigue, which often is "remedied" with further consumption, with more pronounced side effects.

It should be clear that you do not receive energy by drinking coffee, and that the only way to recharge your batteries is by a healthy and proper rest that is in alignment with circadian rhythms.

The same goes for tea and cocoa, albeit less pronounced. However, it is advisable not to consume any of these beverages on a daily basis.

Alternatives to Coffee

Coffee, as already mentioned, has probably been so successful not only for the chemical effects it has, but also because it became a symbol of peaceful coexistence of different people.

During work breaks, as well as in meetings with friends and similar situations, having a coffee has become a sort of obligatory ritual.

Given that, the usual intake is certainly not healthy, there are now many alternatives on the market, in my opinion, even tastier; you can replace the classic black gold cup.

Everyone knows of barley but there are also various mixtures, such as spelt and other grains.

Even chicory coffee, derived from the roots of the plant, is a viable alternative, which also seems to have anti-inflammatory properties.

Also, do not forget about all of the different infusions or tisanes, certainly among the healthiest, and possibly extracts or blended fruit and vegetables.

Finally, it is good to remember not to add any type of sugar to the preparation.

Learn to Walk

Walking is wonderful!

It is a physical activity that promotes relaxation of mind, body and spirit. Walking can be a real panacea for your well-being. Especially if taken in natural environments, rich in vegetation, and far from confusion and traffic.

It is relaxing because it allows you to stay in contact with nature, you can hear the sounds, and experience the scents and colors, but it is also a great way to keep muscles active, strengthen bones and joints, as well as being beneficial to the cardiovascular system.

For those who have specific athletic goals, or at least for those who want to tone up, or improve their body composition, it is not the only activity necessary and sufficient, but to promote a weight loss or at least a maintenance of ideal weight, it remains one of the best possible exercises.

I always advise people to commit to you do. Initially, I suggest you do so at your own pace, choosing a suitable way, possibly in the countryside, hearing the sounds of nature.

Taking pleasure in what you do, will make you passionate about walking, and add it in your daily life.

Humans were born to be in contact with nature, so, when it triggers those instincts, it will probably soon become a regular, if not daily activity.

Find a way to incorporate short walks throughout your day. Perhaps in the morning, evening, and during work breaks, as well as on the weekends when you have more free time.

Walking is pleasant and relaxing, either alone or in company. Periodically, you can organize hiking and small excursions outside the city, to enjoy the abundance that nature can offer with its landscapes and its beauty.

Hiking is really extraordinary and to practice it may cause it to develop into a passion. Perhaps enough to entice you to organize even longer camping excursions in order to fully enjoy the benefits of nature's bounty.

It is important to consider physical activity, or movement in general, as a pleasure.

It is not necessary to over commit, but simply to exploit the moment.

You can also use a pedometer to check your progress, provided its use does not become a craze that defeats the purpose of walking for enjoyment first and foremost.

Insights: Walking After Meals

We have already mentioned how lunch should be considered the main meal of the day.

Eating according to the HND system means avoiding glycemic peaks and the following rebound of hypoglycemia. However, after eating, to encourage digestion,and to feel a little lighter, especially if we have to face other work commitments, a healthy walk is the best solution.

It is important to always be mindful of breathing deeply and completely. Exposing your arms and face to sunlight are great ways to get a good dose of Vitamin D, which is essential to preventative health.

Even after dinner, a long walk is appropriate to facilitate digestion, and to relax your body and muscles in general, in order to promote a good night's rest. For optimal health, it is best for people to stay in motion throughout the day and be sedentary as little as possible. Today, however, many jobs require you to sit for extended periods of time.

What follows is fatigue, including psychological, which then further promotes a sedentary lifestyle in people who, once their work commitments have ended, sit comfortable on sofas or armchairs, attached to the remote control of the television, mobile phones or tablets.

So we find ourselves, at the end of the day, not having passed the 4-5 thousand daily steps, which represent less than half the minimum required!

Adopting small tricks, such as acquiring the habit of walking after lunch, after dinner, and possibly in the morning, as well as creating improvements in well-being and fitness, offers the possibility of feeling more active and efficient, and helps to maintain a constant weight, or a reduction of weight for those who need it.

Breathing

Breathing is a natural act, often overlooked, and is essential to the functioning of our body.

It is said that most people use less than a third of their respiratory capacity.

The quality of your breathing can impact your life on many levels: good breathing helps concentration, relaxation and physical potential. Therefore, learning to manage your breath is crucial to increase your overall well-being.

Inadequate breathing can, hinder the elimination of dangerous toxins that if not disposed of creates stagnant blood in the tissue and harmful oxidation processes.

Physical activity helps to regulate respiratory phases, resulting in substantial benefits.

How to breathe

There are two respiratory acts: inhalation and exhalation.

For further investigation, the breath can be divided into 4 main types:

- HIGH BREATHING: a fast and frequent, shallow breath, which is normally used.

- MEDIUM BREATHING: introduces and emits a greater amount of air (generally found when practicing physical activity).

- DEEP BREATHING: a full breath.

- TOTAL BREATHING: involves the lungs entirely, and also the musculature of the rib cage, the diaphragm in particular.

At certain times of the day, even during meditation (which will be discussed later), it is important to learn how to manage total breathing: the benefits are amazing, both physically and during relaxation and it eliminates stress and tension; it is also an excellent way to help physical and muscle recovery after training or competitions.

Total Breathing improves concentration and psycho-physical efficiency, which is why I consider it to be essential before tackling important commitments, such as tests, examinations or public relation situations. It is also important for athletes as it prepares them for games and competitions.

There are several techniques of deep breathing that are very simple to perform.

One technique works well with meditation:

- Sit in the lotus position, or in any convenient position, but remain aware (do not doze off but be vigilant and present).

- Concentrate and focus on your breathing for at least five minutes.

- Begin to inhale slowly and deeply, to the maximum contraction of the diaphragm, and continue with an equally deep exhalation.

- You can help by placing a hand on the chest, so as to perceive the movements of the respiratory phases that follow one another.

Using this technique for 10-15 minutes a day, constitutes a real practice of well-being, resulting in relaxation and concentration. Take just a quarter hour of your time: you will be surprised by the benefits you will get!

Meditation

Meditation, derives from Latin and means reflection.

It is a method which the HND system strongly recommends to follow in order to savor a deep inner peace, leaving the mind calm and peaceful.

You can apply it to your daily meditation, as a relaxation technique, but I think it is a terrific way to raise awareness and spirituality, and an excellent form of care for oneself.

It is also a useful practice for the body, as it allows you to relax the muscles, often contracted by stress and daily routines.

Meditation allows you to reach a state of fullness and balance, essential for a complete well-being.

How to meditate

No great preparations or special equipment are needed. It is enough to carve out some free time and a place, far from the noise.

The most suitable time is early in the morning. In the afternoon or in the evening it becomes more complicated because of the commitments and the general state of fatigue, in which we find ourselves after a day's work.

Sit in a comfortable position. The lotus position is suggested, with a straight back and eyes closed, preferably on an empty stomach.

You can follow different meditation techniques.I recommend using Vipassana meditation, one of the oldest practiced in India, and based on the observation of the breath.

For the timing, everything depends on the time you have available. It can vary from 10-15 minutes, up to a few hours.

Taking a single course can serve to help understand the basic techniques and to appreciate the first benefits, but it is the continuous practice which is where it is most effective.

Benefits of Meditation

The benefits related to meditation, are tangible in everyday life: greater energy flow, more physical efficiency, greater concentration, ability to better manage stress and control emotions.

Many scientific studies show that the application of meditative techniques have a positive impact on those who are sick. [29,30,31,32]

Meditation helps to restore a state of well-being and balance, because our general state of health is also influenced by our mental and spiritual condition.

Meditating is a training for body, mind and spirit. It is in alignment with food and physical activity as an essential practice to reach maximum well-being and to aid in increasing, day by day, one's awareness.

For these reasons, the HND system emphasizes the importance of meditation, and invites you to practice it constantly in everyday life.

Insights: Yoga

Contrary to what we sometimes hear people say, yoga is neither a religion nor a sport, much less a type of cult.

It is a discipline that connects the body, mind and spirit, in order to help you live better and in harmony with the surrounding world.

Yoga is undoubtedly effective. In fact, there are hundreds of traditions behind this practice.

It originated in India more than two thousand years ago, Since then, styles, methodologies and teaching methods have changed and evolved, but the ultimate goal consisting in achieving a balance between the three dimensions has remained unchanged.

This discipline is in tune with the HND method, because in practice it calls for a healthy lifestyle and an increase in awareness.

To achieve results requires commitment, dedication and perseverance, but also only 15-20 minutes a day may be sufficient to appreciate yoga's benefits.

The results are found in:

- **Physical Benefits:** increased strength, flexibility and balance. Improved function of organs and tissues with detoxification mechanisms from harmful substances. Improvements in breathing and circulation; preventative against problems concerning the spine.

- **Mental Benefits:** reduces anxiety, stress and depression. Promotes the ability to concentrate and clear your mind. It makes people more aware of food choices and lifestyle habits.

With this practice, the body becomes more agile and flexible; concentration on the breath increases the proprioceptive ability and trains the mind to better handle emotional situations of everyday life. With regular exercise you can adjust the flow of energy through chakra control (energy centres of the body), clarifying physical, mental and spiritual issues.

In order to achieve these results, we must remember that yoga makes use of rules and practices to be respected: there are countless positions, including many born in recent years.

There are different types of yoga (Hatha, Ashtanga, Yin, Lyengar, Vinyasa, Anusara, Kundalini, Bikram, Power, Sivananda, etc.), each of which has specific characteristics and different practices, whose ultimate aim is, however, the improvement of the self.

My advice is to inquire about each practice, possibly test lessons to find the way more akin to your character and your needs.

A good teacher and a good environment are important aspects to consider.

Finally, I stress that yoga is a practice accessible to everyone, even for those with physical limitations, since they can adjust its techniques by adapting them appropriately.

Free Mind and Human Relations

It has been shown that environmental factors, associated with a chronic condition of exposure to stressful factors, lead to hyperactivation of the sympathetic nervous system and hypothalamic-pituitary-cortico-urinary axis, with consequent negative effects, also caused by the increase in abdominal (visceral) fat around the waistline; It is known that excessive abdominal fat is closely associated with metabolic changes such as: insulin resistance, reduced glucose tolerance, dyslipidemia and increased blood pressure.

Stress is therefore a danger, not only psychologically, but also physically, because there is a direct correlation with metabolic diseases.

Managing stress, especially in certain environments and work situations is difficult, but possible. You have to commit to spending some time to yourself and do it every day.

Meditation must be part of one's lifestyle: a daily practice that is as important as diet and movement.

A healthy lifestyle cannot ignore the need to share joys, worries, and projects with other people.

Nobody lives on a desert island, we need human relationships.

We know that the society we live in sometimes leads to mistrust, competition, fear or indifference. But having a positive, free and relaxed attitude allows us to enter into a relationship of empathy with others that benefits all involved.

To communicate, it is necessary to listen: putting yourself in an attitude of acceptance and positivity is the first step towards a fulfilling relationship.

It is nice to build close and deep relationships with other people. I suggest tending to a behavior similar to that of children; or to experience events as if for the first time, without taking everything for granted, focusing on listening on pleasant moments, and also appreciating the little things in the world around us.

Living life without too much frenzy, without tending to challenges or unreachable goals, helps people to be calmer, more relaxed and to strengthen their sense of contentment and well-being.

Try to savor as much as possible from life, without precluding anything.

Love, friendships and dreams to pursue, are the real wealth we have that fulfills us. It is important to be mindful of finding the time necessary to cultivate them and to make it a priority equal to that of our work commitments.

Putting work above all else and at the expense of living a full life can degrade one's quality of life. This often results in becoming obsessed with thoughts of problems which then increase stress levels and ultimately lead to the development of diseases.

Therefore, a healthy lifestyle also requires sharing and relationships, fundamental aspects of human nature, which we must nurture with attention and constancy.

PHYSICAL ACTIVITY ACCORDING TO HND METHOD

As explained many times, HND, does not only relate to health and natural nutrition, but is a true lifestyle, that to be called healthy, should also include regular and constant physical activity, balanced according to the objectives, the characteristics and the athletic level of those who practice it.

People who have high levels of physical efficiency showed a lower risk of developing chronic and cardiovascular disease and have a lower mortality rate. [33,34]

Physical activity is aimed at promoting growth and body function. Besides being an excellent protective instrument, it is also considered an essential therapeutic component in curing diseases. [35]

It is generally preferable to engage in various activities, so as to train all muscle groups and different metabolic systems (aerobic, anaerobic lactic acid, anaerobic alactacid) of the body.

Functional Training in HND

Walking or jogging performed at low intensity, as well as all those exercises performed in the gym using isotonic machines are useful methods to keep active and as prevention against metabolic diseases related to a sedentary lifestyle. But do not represent the most effective means of training as well as amateur sports practices, such as football, running, cycling, basketball or tennis.

Functional training allows you to receive the motor integrity benefits made from natural movements such as running, jumping, and sprinting that was lost due to a system with physical inactivity and that over time has created significant worsening in the motor skills of individuals. [36]

If we think that different people have to resort to drugs and weeks of recovery, simply from lifting a shopping bag, or for playing a match of football with friends, you can see that it is necessary to take action to recover the physical strength needed not only to carry out daily chores, but also to increase wellness, efficiency and health conditions.

For adequate physical preparation it is recommended to perform exercises standing, with bursts of motion, changing direction and the use of free weights in order also to enhance the neuromuscular system.

Everything must be customized depending on the subject, but in general, when we talk about physical activity, it is necessary to increase the intensity, then the effort, in order to obtain an improvement of the functional capacity. [37]

Non challenging exercises, often carried out by sitting or lying down, are not adequate for the objective.

The HND method suggests as a basis, movement and an active lifestyle, but also includes a workout in phases, programmed properly and aimed not only at physical efficiency, but also prevention. This is especially true as we age, when small injuries require a large recovery time and simple everyday distractions can also be fatal (just think of how debilitating a ruptured femur can be in the elderly).

Training Goals

Several times in this book, I stressed that health is closely related to physical activity and movement. So it is easy to see that the goal of physical activity and sports in general, must be to safeguard health.

It is good to know that physical activity can and should be practiced at any age and in any physical and metabolic condition, of course adapted to each individual.

Only 30 minutes a day of moderate to intense activity is enough to significantly reduce the risk of the onset of chronic degenerative diseases that plague the Western world. [38,39]

Exercising also improves one's physique and so their aesthetic appearance, delaying the aging process. [40]

You can exercise for several reasons: one of these is constituted by the desire to improve performance in order to compete or engage in some type of sport. Even so, training for the sheer pleasure of it is the goal, as it brings satisfaction, creates energy and vitality, and helps to relieve stress and tension.

Physical Activities, How Much And When Do It

In the course of daily activities, plan to devote at least three times a week to real training sessions: it is good to distinguish movement from working out.

Movement, which may be walking, or any of those activities that are carried out in a dynamic way that don't involve excessive stress to the body, are also an essential parameter and can be considered a baseline of regular daily activity.

Humans are born to be active and inherently want to maintain or improve their own condition of wellness. In order to achieve that goal, it is necessary to keep moving throughout the day. Exercising on the other hand, is substantially different, in that it is a movement precisely programmed in order to achieve certain physical and metabolic objectives.

For example, you can exercise to increase muscle mass, improve strength, resistance and speed or simply to achieve a certain level of cardiovascular fitness as a preventive measure.

According to the HND method, the movement is as important as exercise, but to be more precise, it can be said that while the movement and being active are a part of human nature, exercise, although useful, is not indispensable.

Surely, a person involved in a physical activity, structured and planned, aimed at a certain specific objective, enjoys significant advantages over those who do not.

All subjects can exercise: from young to old those with diseases to those who have suffered trauma or injury, of course, with modifications and depending on the desired outcome and abilities of the participants. The workout will differ greatly between one who is interested in increasing cardiovascular fitness from that of a senior who needs to strengthen their bone structure.

Each person needs both a preventive and performance level of a specific program of physical activity that should take one's lifestyle into consideration.

You cannot offer the same type of workout to a person who wants to run a marathon, compared to one who performs strenuous work.

The first rule, therefore, is to follow a program that will achieve the desired physical outcomes.

Physical activity, as such, results in a production of stress and free radicals, which when not classified in a particular context, can sometimes be very harmful to the individual.

The purpose of the activity should be to create a benefit and not harm. So if you do not know the chosen activity well, much less your body, it is always advisable to seek help from an expert in the field you are interested in exploring.

Three workouts per week is a good start in general terms. It is assumed that an athlete wishing to try a particular sport will have different needs than that of an amateur.

What must be clear is that the weekly activity program should also include recovery days in order to give the body a chance to benefit from the work done and grow stronger from it.

The weekly frequency of training also varies according to the type of activity that takes place: strength training requires more recovery time than routine activities such as jogging. This will allow the affected muscles to recover properly.

The frequency of workouts also varies according to age, as older people may require longer recovery periods.

As for the time of day, contrary to the claims by various experts, training should be done in the late afternoon rather than early morning. It should not interfere with the eliminative phases of the body but instead allow the body to complete its morning detoxification process.

Working out in the morning does not guarantee good performance and it seems to increase the production of free radicals.

In the evening the hormonal levels are such as to promote anabolism and muscle growth, as they have high levels of testosterone and low cortisol. Also the body temperature is higher then and improves athletic performance due to the great benefits that are created with warmed up muscles and joints.

Obviously, it is not advisable to exercise too late, since the production of lactic acid, combined with DOMS (post exercise muscle pain), may interfere with the success of sleep. It should be added that training later implies eating later, therefore altering the rules of the circadian rhythms.

Summary

- *Define the objective of the training*

- *Program the frequency and volume of training by: goals, age, job, lifestyle in general.*

- *Do not exceed and do not overdo activities to the point where the damage outweighs the benefits.*

- *Train in the late afternoon to take advantage of optimal physical and metabolic conditions.*

General Physical Preparation

Before you engage in any physical activity, especially of a certain intensity, you need to "warm up" your body to prepare it for an increase in motion.

This will aid in a creating a resistance to fatigue, thereby improving the recovery time.

The warm-up can be of varying lengths depending on the physical condition of the subject.

To obtain benefits is necessary increase the intensity of effort. For example, with a sprint or progressions if we are talking about running, will reduce recovery times: creating circuits of exercises, with or without increasing intensities, is a very effective method to increase the resistance to fatigue. [36, 37]

HND Circuit

The HND circuit constitutes a highly effective method for weight loss and at the same time toning tissues: HND is the base of the system and constitutes a convenient and fast workout that can be done anywhere.

The HND circuit consists of carrying out a series of exercises in sequence (circuit training), using different muscle groups of the body.

Each exercise is done by following a certain number of repetitions (usually 10-12 reps) or seconds (30-60 seconds etc.) with the speed and intensity programmed according to the desired results, and without rest periods between one station and another.

At the end of the sequence of exercises, the circuit can be repeated several times, depending on the intensity level that you want to achieve.

The HND circuit presents some basic features:

- Use of free weights or bodyweight alone.

- Exercises basically carried out by "standing".

- Multi-joint exercises (that involving large muscle groups).

- Good intensity and speed of execution.

You can work both in time and/or with a precise number of reps.

The circuit may provide different exercise stations, but is also possible to opt for example, to a program of 2 mini circuits of 4 stations each, one of which is used for the purpose of increasing the overall warmup and one as the real workout.

In regard to the recovery time, theoretically you do not have pauses between one exercise and the next, but you can opt for approximately 1-2 minutes of rest at the end of each circuit and before starting the next round.

Start with the lower body (such as a squat or a deadlift, performed on different types of equipment or scenarios), followed by an exercise for the upper body, incorporating those larger muscle groups, as the dorsal, pectorals and deltoids.

It is important to remember not to do exercises that "isolate" small muscle groups (such as a curl for biceps) as multi-joint exercises, such as bench press, is a full exercise for different muscle groups, (mainly pectorals, triceps and anterior deltoid) and not only relates to an isolated beam.

When the body moves, in fact, different muscle groups act in sync, thereby performing complex exercises involving multiple joints, it means train and play gestures and everyday situations.

Once the technique is executed properly, it should be fast and explosive in order to improve neuromotor abilities.

The choice of using free weights by "standing" facilitates the most muscle coordination while at the same time reinforcing the stabilizing muscles that assist in the movement.

The use of free weights improves the synchronization of the movements, strengthening the joints and helping the body to absorb external forces.

It is important to train all of the muscles in a balanced way: muscle imbalances can often lead to injuries and may cause the body to develop out of proportion.

It is necessarily expected thrust and traction exercises with the limitation of the exercises of flexion-extension that generally limit the movement to a single articulation.

As mentioned above it is important to recreate the habitual motions used in everyday life. So it's good to perform standing exercises such as lifting weights from the ground and pushing them over the head. This exercise improves posture and agility, avoiding the risk of accidents and problems that may occur with the simple lifting of a grocery bag.

Before starting circuit training, you need to warm up well and appropriately and according to the heating protocol explained in the section.

You can complete the warm up with exercises for the abs or at least for the core training for a comprehensive and diversified training.

Types of Exercises and Equipment

For effective results, as mentioned, you should perform exercises that involve various muscle groups, and so, more joints.

These types of exercises are more complex, as they require good coordination and good neuromuscular skill. However, they are far more effective than single joint exercises, as there is a real commitment of the nervous system in conjunction with the stabilizer muscles.

Listed below are the basic training exercises, divided into works of push and pull, which are useful in achieving a harmonious and balanced development of the body: with a push exercise, it is always advisable to include its complimentary pull exercise..

- **Lower Body Push:** squats (front and back), pistol squats, lunges and variants

- **Lower Body Pull:** deadlifts, turn and tear (the most advanced)

- **Upper Body Push:** bench presses, slow forward, pushups, dip to parallel.

- **Upper Body Pull:** rower, chins

Remember that from these basic exercises, you can create an infinite number of variations, using both body weight alone and with the help of fitness equipment.

Varying the modality and the type of tool helps to make the workout addictive, avoiding the monotony that could take over in the long term.

If for example you decide to perform a squat, that is face-to-free body, with the aid of a TRX, with a barbell, with a Kettlebell, with a wall-ball or other, is irrelevant, because the biomechanics of execution is the same and the loads or turns repetitions, support the objective.

Practical Examples (Free Body or With Weights)

CIRCUIT 1

- Squat

- Row

- Deadlift with one leg

- Military press

CIRCUIT 2

- Front Lunge

- Push-up

- Deadlift

- Pull up

VARIATIONS

Inside each circuit you can add exercises for the abdominals and lower back (especially for beginners), which serve to increase the recovery time

- Squat

- Row

- **Crunch**

- Deadlift with one leg

- Military press

- Lower back (lumbar)

For the more advanced you can increase the difficulty by inserting dynamic exercises (such as with the use of a kettlebell)

- Squat

- **Swing with KB**

- Row

- **Swing with KB**

- Deadlift with one leg

- **Swing with KB**

- Military press

- **Swing with KB**

Abdominal and lumbar are widely encouraged, but it may also be performed during the warm up.

Increase the Difficulty

Training needs change over time to be effective so you need to act on the volume and intensity.

- **Volume total**: it is sufficient increase the number of exercises or laps of the circuit (from 2 to 3, from 3 to 4, and so on). Also, increase the number of repetitions or the duration of each exercise (keeping the load unchanged).

- **Intensity**: the training weight (increases from 10 to 12 kg for example) or the speed of execution. Also reducing the recovery time results in an increase of intensity.

Run Training

To achieve incredible physical improvements in my HND system my advice to combine the HND circuits of strength-resistance, workouts targeted to cardiovascular fitness and of various metabolic systems (aerobic, anaerobic lactose and anaerobic alactacid).

In this text I considered running as a routine activity that can be done anywhere without any special equipment.

Any other endurance sports, such as cycling, swimming, cross-country skiing, skating, rowing, etc., can also be taken into account for equally effective results and aimed at the achievement of the same objectives.

There are many benefits of running, not only as a preventive way to keep in shape, but also to liberate the mind from stress and promote a positive state of mind.

Running is also useful for strengthening the immune system, in that it increases up to six times the production of killer white blood cells and interferon. [41, 42]

For those who are overweight or not used to running, I recommend limiting, at least in the first period, their activity to walking, and alternating fast walking: surely it is less effective than running, but will avoid joint and bone damage. We have to remember that running has an "air time", where both limbs are off the ground. Therefore, the impact with the ground in heavy people can cause excessive impact, caused by the force of gravity. The same applies to those who have never run. Plantar support and the overall biomechanics of running may result in damage and injuries, perhaps serious, at joints. My advice for beginners then is to be monitored an expert at least in the initial phase, because learning proper athletic form is crucial to maintaining the correct technique.

Regarding training, I recommend scheduling days for low intensity runs, alternating with runs comprised of intermittent sprints, progressively or as repetitions, and scheduled according to the desired achieved outcome.

Even the fartlek or a continuous run where they are introduced at random (without routine) changes of rhythm, may fall into the method of the alternating run.

The continuing run is more suitable as a recovery phase: the capillary vasodilation, created by the athletic gesture, promotes the greater perfusion then the oxygenation of the muscles and the elimination of toxins, allowing a more rapid and efficient recovery.

For those that are physically active and receptive to that lifestyle, I advise including some sporting activities.

If you like running, it can be found to be relaxing, especially if practiced in natural environments such as parks or forests.

The interval run instead consists of a real workout, aiming to improve conditional abilities (strength, endurance and speed), as well as cardiovascular fitness.

With interval running you can obtain maximum exertion levels . The thing is to always respect the training principles and increase the reps or gradual intensity with adequate recovery times between one session and the next: two running interval workouts per week are more than enough, even for an athlete who aspires to do some kind of amateur competition.

Combining running with the HND strength/endurance circuits appears to be ideal for people who are overweight and intend to lose weight fast.

How to Build an Interval Training

After a suitable warm up you can start the real workout phase, always starting from 10-15 minutes of gentle running, in order to raise the body temperature for a better performance and to avoid possible injuries.

You can proceed essentially in 3 ways:

- **Time:** progression, sprint or at least the rhythm variation is measured in a very precise time interval, ranging from 5 seconds up to 5-10 minutes and more, depending on the objectives. The recovery between a variation and the next, in this case, is incomplete (the heart rate does not return to basal levels). The method is a good workout, especially for the heart and its size, elasticity, as well as for the various metabolic mechanisms, related to the use of glucose.

- **Distance:** the intensity increment is defined in a precise distance (e.g. 50 meters, 200 meters, 400 meters, etc.). In these cases the recovery is complete (the heart rate is returned to basal levels). It is a workout protocol, especially to increase the running speed.

- **Fartlek:** variation of rhythm is performed randomly without considering time or distance, so it will always be different: an overpass, a tree, a road sign, a small hill are all reference points that can be considered during a fartlek. It usually follows a regular route, creating rhythm changes according to the references taken. These changes of rhythm are generally quite short (usually no more than a minute). The recovery is incomplete, therefore, the objectives are roughly the same as the first type (timed workouts).

You can create different workouts and, especially for athletes wishing to engage in agonism, there are well-defined protocols, quite challenging to achieve the desired results.

In our case we do not run for any purpose, other than to have fun and to differentiate the workout, trying at the same time to make it effective.

Practical Examples

Time

- Warm up

- Every minute of jogging, sprint of 10 seconds (20 minutes total)

- Recovery

Distance

- Warm up

- 5x 400 meters, maximum speed (2' recovery between sets)

- Recovery

Fartlek

- Circuit of 5 km hilly, variable sprints at each slope increase (es.

- Overpass, off, climb, etc.).

Planning the Week

To obtain noticeable results and maintain them, my advice first and foremost is to exercise consistently and with pleasure.

Everyone can plan their week as they see fit but try to respect the principles of training: if in the winter season (due to the cold, a few hours of light, etc.) you are less likely to engage in running, you can replace it with any other activity, predominantly of an aerobic type:

swimming, boating, biking or skating but also hiking and walks (especially if performed in mountainous terrain and for a long time) are all excellent alternatives; the winter months are ideal to organize hiking and excursions with family, friends or even alone.

In principle, two circuit workouts with overload and 2 running sessions (or similar activities) are more than enough to achieve a good level of fitness, improving wellness and physical fitness.

Beginners can start with two or three workouts per week, while the more advanced should not have any problem with doing 5-6 sessions per week. It is good to remember that it is not the number that makes the difference, as the quality and type of exercise being performed.

The planned rest days can vary depending on the physical state of the person: if you have planned a workout, but you are very tired for various reasons it is useless to force oneself to train, because it would be counterproductive. Better to rest or take a long walk, to relax and defuse the accumulated tensions. Here's an example:

Training Week	Beginner	Advanced
Monday	Rest	Circuit
Tuesday	Circuit	Slow Run
Wednesday	Rest	Rest
Thursday	Run	Circuit
Friday	Rest	Run
Saturday	Slow Run	Rest
Sunday	Rest	Run

Remember to always be active and that a walk can and should be included in the daily workout schedule

LOSE WEIGHT WITH HND METHOD

T*he increase of weight does not consist only in an esthetic problem but, as we have seen, is the cause of physical and metabolic consequences also quite serious, especially if protracted.*

With the HND method you will finally have the possibility of losing weight effectively and rapidly while preserving the results achieved over time.

No matter how many attempts and how many failures you have had in life, the HND method will enable you to reach your goals!

Food for Weight Loss

It is always said that having a CALORIC DEFICIT (energy consumption greater than addition), was the only method needed for slimming. This has given rise to a misconception (see the special section of the body composition, p. 9) that simply implementing any low-calorie diet will get results. As we have seen, weight loss actually exists, but mainly at the expense of lean body mass, with a likely gaining of weight in the medium to long term (fat and not lean muscle mass). With HND, it is not necessary to make any type of caloric restrictions.

As we have already seen, low-calorie diets are often the cause of secondary effects of the yo-yo type, with not only regaining the initial weight lost, but a subsequent additional weight increase.

When a body is well nourished, it will automatically start the purification processes and slimming.

Excess fat is a consequence of eating poorly, so by balancing the diet, the body will automatically respond by eliminating all of that unnecessary excess.

Detox Phase

As a start, my advice is for two to four weeks to focus on purifying your body, stimulating the elimination of waste and toxic substances, placing the body in the best position to start the slimming process.

The digestive system is full of waste, toxins and mucus. Sedimentation in the intestinal wall inhibits the proper absorption of nutrients and hinders the various metabolic processes of elimination in the body.

In essence, at the basis of weight gain is almost always a strong state of toxicity.

With a diet rich in fruits and soup or vegetable purée, acts directly on this issue restoring the correct functioning of the digestive and metabolic processes of the body.

Example of detox phase

(This is just an example, everything must be seen and customized according to the season and the patient's eating habits).

- **Breakfast**: 3 oranges (or aqueous fresh fruit)

- **Snack**: 2 bananas

- **Lunch**: generous bowl of seasonal leafy vegetables and avocado with lemon juice, followed by a plate of cold potatoes with herbs and spices

- **Snack**: 2 red apples (or fresh fruit salad)

- **Dinner**: vegetables purée and potatoes with hemp and sunflower seeds

There may be more or less drastic detox phases; remember that the program should be customized according to the individual.

What should be clear is that it is only a phase, which is necessary to restore the baseline condition of the subject.

You can also avoid this transitional phase, immediately applying the regular phase of the Healthy Natural Diet, with the only difference being to slow down the processes of weight loss in the first period.

How Much You Should Come Down

There is not a definite number of kilograms to be determined because this is not a race, so each has their own route to follow.

Weight loss, in fact, is affected by the initial weight of the subject, age, medical history, eating habits and lifestyles.

Average weight loss is around one kg per week for men and 700/800g for women.

There are also higher weight losses, especially in the initial phases in those subjects that start from a severe water imbalance.

The decline in these cases is not only due to fat loss, but at the elimination of excess fluids containing waste substances accumulated in the interstitial spaces.

By restoring balance in the body, it moves to reactivating the purifying capacity, hampered by time, which can then return to performing its intended function, and then allows the fast removal of excess fluid.

Headaches, Fatigue and Intestinal Problems

It can happen especially in the initial phases of the Healthy Natural Diet, or during the Detox phase, of having problems such as fatigue, headaches and sometimes diarrhea or intestinal problems.

It is a normal condition in that the body in the eliminative phase, expels toxins or at least those harmful residues, from time sedimented in various tissues.

The waste products from the tissue transfer to the blood: the more a person turns out to be "toxic", the more likely that these symptoms occur.

The same thing applies in the intestine, where the sedimented material on the walls is eliminated in the form of diarrhea or otherwise feces not formed and malodorous.

Maintenance Phase

After an initial detox phase, the maintenance diet stays the same as the standard HND program. It will probably be necessary, over time, to increase the food intake for the body to function properly, and to have the muscular benefits. If there is not enough food, muscle growth will be inhibited.

It is not the amount of food that makes you fat, but the nutritional quality, so unnatural foods are of no use to our metabolic systems: if you focus on quality, hunger/satiety signals automatically take over according to the requirements of the body and without confusion as to how to metabolize "empty calories.".

Often, when we eat high quantities of food with little nutritional value it causes our body to experience a delayed response time to knowing when we have eaten enough. This can often lead to unpleasant consequences related to digestion that can result in discomfort and abdominal swelling for prolonged periods. This does not happen if you consume quality foods that are nutrient dense. Instead, satiety occurs gradually and is noticeable, without problems, and without over eating.

Excess fat is not natural for our bodies, as a result, if you eat and train properly, it is very easy and weight loss is quick.

Physical Activity: How Much and What

Physical activity is essential in the slimming process. To lose weight and do it effectively, it is understood that you have to avoid a sedentary lifestyle. This in turn means that you must have an active lifestyle while following a natural and healthy diet plan, such as the Healthy Natural Diet.

A common mistake is thinking that with walking alone significant weight loss can be achieved. Walking is a good foundation to engage in on a daily basis, but to be physically fit will require more effort.

Another common misconception is the belief that to promote weight loss, the addition of aerobic activity rather than High Intensity Interval Training (HIIT) is the preferred choice. Even here, there is no scientific evidence to confirm this theory, on the contrary, constant activity such as a long jog, which would be considered moderate activity over time, is subject to metabolic adaptations that lead to the muscles involved burning less as they adapt to the activity. Moreover, improvements in muscle mass also decrease over time because they are no longer adequately stressed by the redundant activity level. Combine this with a low calorie diet and there is a reduction of musculature and therefore, of metabolism. Running also, does not produce significant benefits over the other muscle groups of the body, which will remain only slightly toned. This is yet another reason that it is not a very effective activity in terms of energy consumption. [36]

According to the HND method, repeated anaerobic efforts with incomplete recovery are much more effective than a continuous activity, as they provide more stress to the muscles, generating metabolism increases, which will also go on for several hours after the session.

High Intensity training avoids muscle adaptation, and in every training session you must create the conditions for the growth and improvement of muscle tone and reflexes.

In addition to training at high intensity, one must consider several bands and muscle groups, then a workout that involves the whole body (total body) to favour metabolic increases even in the less stressed musculature every day.

High intensity training means an increase in the post-exercise oxygen consumption (EPOC), which will lead to fat burning (afterburn) long after the exercise is completed (fat is the fuel that is consumed mostly at rest). [43,44,45]

So, rather than create a caloric deficit, the focus should be on increasing fat consumption, which is achieved by increasing the rest oxygen consumption.

Do not forget too, that it is the muscles that consume energy (fat) and as a result, a well-trained muscle (in this case more well-trained muscles) determines a higher fat consumption.

The most suitable workout to get effective results in a short time is the HND circuit (you can also create 5-10 minute circuits).

The circuit must be done with a certain criterion (explained in detail in the section), but it is also possible to opt for mixed circuits with overload exercises, combined with sprints or circuits only focused on them.

Increasing the intensity avoids muscle adaptations and allows for constant improvements.

It is good to remember to always establish a schedule of workouts that includes periods of "discharge" and muscle recovery: circuit training is short but very intense, so it is appropriate to include a day of rest between workouts, or every two workouts for more advanced athletes.

In the days of rest if you still want to remain active. Perhaps a long walk or a continuous run (about 45 minutes) to help the oxygenation of the muscles and improve cardiovascular fitness.

It is important to introduce oxygenation sections not only to create benefits to the microcirculation, but also because they are very useful in eliminating toxins or waste substances that can accumulate in the tissues.

Running is also a good therapy for relaxation and unloading stress as well as nervous tension.

Organize and Program Physical Exercise

Exercises carried out for weight loss, not only promote an increase of metabolism able to eliminate excess fat, but are also necessary in allowing the development of proper muscle tone, which is an essential consideration in the case of heavy weight loss. Maintaining a high energy level will also keep the metabolic mechanisms for eliminating fat working more efficiently. [46]

Physical activity must be programmed, differentiated and at adequate levels and frequencies in that, an excess of activity could be dangerous not only for health reasons, but especially for the slimming process.

High volumes of exercise, excessive in relation to usual movements, force the body to a disproportionate workload which significantly increases in the basal metabolic rate.

High intensity training with its high energy expenditure must be compensated for in some way. The only way that the body has to compensate for this is with the intake of food, especially sugar, because muscles not used to training hard require a significantly higher energy expenditure than muscles trained to do so.

If we do not follow the general rules of sports nutrition, circadian cycles and the basic principles of healthy eating, it is very easy to indulge in and overeat foods of poor nutritional quality.

It is common practice for individuals who engage in certain amateur sports, who work out at particular times such as lunchtime, late evening or early morning, creating imbalances around circadian cycles, meal management or hours of sleep.

These situations, if not controlled properly, won't help in achieving the desired results and will often sabotage them.

For this reason, it is always better to not improvise anything. Before undertaking any activity, you need to implement careful planning and possibly get help from qualified professionals in order to not only prepare adequately, but also to optimize the exercises and work schedules.

Change the Training

It is also important to vary the type of training to not create physical and metabolic adaptations, then defeat the slimming processes as well as improvement of muscle tone.

The change of workouts basically means two things:

1. **Working on the total training amount, intensity or recovery periods of the same type of sport:** for example, if today I trained for 30 minutes and the next session I will train 40 minutes, I created an increase in the amount of training. If today I did 400 meter reps with 1 minute rests between reps, and the next session I do the same number of reps with shorter breaks, I have reduced the recovery time and so increased the intensity that way. In this way you can achieve positive results without changing the type of sport.

2. **Change the type of sport:** in this case we change the athletic movement and work different muscle groups. This type of cross training is just as important in the metabolic and slimming purposes. Of course, it is always better to play sports rather different from each other: for example, swimming and cycling, rather than running and combat sports. Biking and skating, for example, are as effective together because they work the same muscle groups.

How Much To Workout for Effective Weight Loss

The frequency of the various training sessions depends on the characteristics of the person.

Exercising too much, and too often, does not appear to be effective either for weight loss, muscle growth, or even overall health.

Having low recovery periods, especially for subjects not conditioned means creating a hard and stressful situation as well as the excessive production of free radicals.

On average, the ideal solution consists of 3 to 4 training sessions per week, 30 to 50 minutes per session, with at least one day of rest between one workout and the next.

However, every day you need to walk to avoid a sedentary lifestyle.

Training For Strength and Hypertrophy.

The HND circuits and interval training are very effective for the weight loss process because, if done properly and with incremental overload, help to preserve, and in some cases (especially in untrained subjects), to increase muscle mass.

The HND circuits, despite the use of overload, are classified as resistance training (strength development over time), so in the long term, people who do not follow proper recovery and lead a rather stressful lifestyle, risk weakening the muscles which then lower your metabolism, and eventually defeat the slimming process and create a type of "deadlock" phase.

In these cases, the most common thought may be to increase physical activity ("I'm not losing weight, so I have to increase the workout"). In fact, often you must do the opposite: increase the recovery time and enter into a "static" exercise phase aimed at developing strength and hypertrophy, to increase muscle mass.

The exercises to be carried out are almost the same as those used for the HND circuits (see p. 111), then multi-joint exercises with free weights alternating pushing and pulling work; change only the mode of execution.

Among the tools the barbell is the most effective (for achieving high loads).

Remember that these guidelines are valid, especially for active people, who perform at least 3-4 workouts per week and who have more training experience.

For those that are sedentary or with less time available, the execution of HND circuits, alternating running or walking is already more than enough to ensure improvements and the achievement of one's objectives (albeit perhaps more slowly).

Strength, Hypertrophy and Training Mode

There are several definitions of muscle strength:

-   "Muscle strength can be defined as the ability that the intimate components of muscle matter have to contract, in the practice of shortening". (Vittori)

-   "Strength is the ability of skeletal muscle to produce tension in various manifestations." (Verchosanskij)

-   "You can define the strength of a man as his ability to defeat an external resistance or oppose with a muscular effort." (Zaciorrskij)

It can be said that, the starting point of any motor activity, results from strenght: the greater the strenght, the greater the speed, resistance, power, etc. Consequently, also the hypertrophy development, which is an increase in muscle volume, may be in some way related to the strenght.

During the year, therefore, in order to safeguard and increase muscle mass, schedule at least 2 training cycles dedicated to these two motor skills.

Strenght: 3-week program with 3 weekly sessions

Load: 85-95% of the RM (repetition maximum).

Repetitions: 3-4

Series: 4-6 per exercise.

Recovery: from 3 to 5 minutes.

Hypertrophy: following a 3-week program with 3-4 weekly sessions

Load: 7 -85% of the RM (repetition maximum).

Repetitions: 6-8

Series: 4-6 per exercise.

Recovery: from 2 to 3 minutes.

Example of Training (barbell)

- SQUAT

- ROW

- DISTENSIONS ABOVE THE HEAD

During the days of recovery, you should walk and make them long walks, or do 30-40 minutes of light running or jogging to facilitate the recovery and oxygenation of muscle tissue.

After each cycle of strength and hypertrophy it is always advisable to include a week of active rest (you can do something light, but it's good to let the muscles rest properly in order to optimize the work done).

Insights: The Crossfit

Lately it has been in vogue to practice this type of activity in gyms and fitness centers.

Without judging the sport itself, beautiful as it may be, remember that this activity, which has its origins in California, is designed for advanced athletes with a certain background of experience.

In today's gyms, we see inexperienced people trying these high-impact sports, often resulting in serious consequences.

Problems at the shoulder joint and rotator cuff are on the top of the list, as well as the spine, followed by muscle trauma and at the joints generally. Not everyone can practice the same sport, needs are different: some need to be faster, stronger or more flexible.

Moreover, these centers are sometimes managed by persons not properly trained.

Crossfit is a sport that should be learned and used wisely, and should be avoided altogether if you have no particular expertise or do not have the perfect execution techniques.

It is more appropriate to start with a functional training, aimed at learning and improving performance techniques without risking damage to the body.

HND Guidelines in Weight Loss

We have seen how important nutrition, physical activity and movement are in general to achieve effective weight loss without incurring damage or problems for the body.

We will now summarize the **guidelines** for effective weight loss according to the HND method.

- **Follow the rules and principles of the Healthy Natural Diet**

- **Provide an initial "detox" phase in order to restore balance and speed up the slimming process**

- Adopt an active lifestyle

- Walk daily and make them long walks

- Do one or more physical activities, properly planned and carried out

- Include an interval training method

- *Workouts both with overloads and running must be total body (overall workouts not just isolated muscle groups).*

- *High intensity HND circuits are useful in the promotion of metabolic consumption and post-exercise oxygen (EPOC).*

- *Do not neglect the required periods of recovery and muscle relaxation*

- *Continue running/jogging sessions to support recovery as well as muscle and tissue oxygenation*

- *Periodically do specific programs devoted to strength and hypertrophy in order to promote muscle growth*

- *Differentiate and always vary the exercises and workouts*

- *Adopt an HND diet, possibly increasing the quantity of food. The secret to losing weight is never be hungry!*

Insights: Localized Weight Loss

This too is a hot topic of contention. I have heard, among other absurdities, of a certain fad fitness programs that claim they have the ability to spot reduce fat in problem areas! Incredible, right? The craziest thing about it is that people buy them!

Localized fat reduction is unrealistic, but solving the problem is simpler than you think.

Our body accumulates fat that is usually deposited in the abdominal (visceral) area for men and that of the buttocks and hips for women.

There are also different genetic tendencies for which there are people whose fat distribution with wind up with more in the legs rather than calves, arms and so on. But this is simply a function of genetics set from birth or in the first years of life, when the body assumes physical features which will remain unchanged in normal weight conditions for the rest of its life.

But we must distinguish the features that are characteristic of the individual (a bit like the color of the eyes or skin) from fat gained due to an unhealthy lifestyle.

In this second case the solution is, the fat gained in those specific points mentioned above, is also what will probably be "burned off" and used for energy during the slimming process.

After that, if there are still aspects of your body you want to improve, you need to incorporate physical activity.

In the HND method the concept of physical activity to take action on these points is based on the principle of blood circulation. In other words, the more the blood circulates in certain sectors, the more favorable conditions will be created for improving the tone of the tissue, eliminating these "problem spots" over time.

Blood, in fact, is the essential nourishment for the tissues. Most of these are vascularised, so the greater the ability to remove fats, also improves the body's ability to remove toxins and various other wastes that accumulate over time.

In the chapter of physical activity, I talked about high-intensity circuits with "displacement" of blood flow from the lower areas of the body to high ones and vice versa.

These are among the most suitable exercises to help improve the profile and the tone of certain parts of your body.

The same is true for food: the HND diet is able to completely purify the body by eliminating waste and sediments stagnated there over time, due at years of poor nutrition; favoring therefore a greater fluidity of the blood and an improved blood perfusion at the periphery or otherwise micro-capillary level, confers a strong nutritional power to the tissues.

To obtain accurate results you need to be consistent over time: weekly or monthly measures will not achieve the desired results.

Beauty Treatments in Localized Slimming

Today, there are many very popular treatments that, in the opinion of those who propose them, would seem to have several effects: the reduction of fat mass, tightening of tissues; from the elimination of cellulite to localized fat reduction.

In this regard, some serious intervention exists, but we must remember that any lasting changes are only possible if created from the inside out.

What's important for our body needs to be done by us and not someone else: eat healthy, do any physical activity and follow an active lifestyle, according to the principles of the Healthy Natural Diet.

The rest is just business and propaganda: the objective is to sell. Various treatments are promoted as a miracle for the external and for the aesthetics, without considering the negative effects.

Shortcuts and miracles do not exist and as I said, you have to do it to get it!

Many people waste time and money chasing fantasies when with simple changes in habits they could get more rewarding and healthy results.

Now, I do not want to lump everything together. I think much progress has been made in this area, but you can intervene only after changing your own habits, improving the ones that are the pillars of a healthy lifestyle: nutrition and physical activity.

No need to beautify a house until you have built the foundation!

With only 4 weeks of the HND method, I am confident that you will be pleasantly surprised by the results. This is just the beginning of a wonderful journey that will take you to an incredible state of health and wellness.

Summary

- We have a genetic physiognomy seat from birth.

- It is not possible to spot reduce fat in problem areas.

- You lose fat in areas of the body the same way that you gained it.

- You can improve physical features of the body, especially if due to incorrect habits.

- To improve nutrition and physical activity it's necessary to be consistent.

- The HND system provides natural nutrition and high intensity circuit training in opposite body areas.

- Supplements and special substances are not necessary.

- Beauty treatments when performed correctly, can help, but only if accompanied with healthy eating and physical activity.

Insights: Training Fasting

According to some myths, the most effective way to lose weight is working out first thing in the morning before eating, thereby: conducting activity with a sugar deficit so that , the body would be "obliged" to burn fat as an energy source.

A full night's rest can consume over 60% of glycogen stores making it easy to train without eating, running out the last stores of sugars and acting on fat metabolism.

It would seem to be a good solution, if not for the little scientific validity of this theory that, in reality, does not show the desired effects. [47,48]

As already mentioned, fats are the fuel that our body gives priority to in low-intensity workouts and this happens whether we ate or not, so the fat consumption is exactly the same in the two conditions. The difference is that if you exercise on an empty stomach, at high intensity, you may compromise the activity due to weakness and fatigue, especially if this is carried out for an extended period of time. [49]

For activities less than an hour in duration, you have to remember that there are still the muscle glycogen stores, because the glycogen used in the night's rest is mainly of hepatic origin. [49]

It is therefore not correct to say that without introducing food, you entered directly into the training situation in a fasting state (sugars derived from muscle glycogen, biochemically speaking, are the same that come for a meal).

If you are not familiar with the early warnings of hypoglycemia, the body may respond with different physical problems such as headaches, weakness, blurred vision and fainting, all of which are not useful for either performance or health.

Additionally, training continued in a sugar shortage condition also has a catabolic effect on muscle mass, increasing the risk of overtraining. [50]

Summary

The fasting training does not lead to faster weight loss, because the consumption of fat is identical with the same intensity and time, compared to a workout done under "normal" condition.

Exercising on an empty stomach can be dangerous for non-adapted people, but also for those who perform long or intense workouts.

Fasting while training or competing may, however, be useful in some situations, especially in running activities when the intestines are particularly sensitive to digestive mechanisms due to the introduction of food: if the activity has a maximum duration of 1.5 hours, do not consume food. It does not particularly influence the performance at the metabolic level, rather, the performance could be better because the digestion process takes away from the precious blood that instead would be sent to the muscle mass.

Sometimes, especially in people who do not have much free time, working out in the early morning is the only possible solution if you want to carry out regular and consistent physical activity.

Having a small breakfast means triggering the digestive processes that impede training, consequently, it is easier to train without eating. So eat a regular breakfast upon completion of the activity (which generally hardly lasts for more than one hour). Again, fasting becomes useful to the cause.

Other Objectives of Training

We have seen how to maintain a healthy state of wellness, physical activity is essential, as well as for weight loss. Circuit training with high intensity and incomplete recovery exercises, together result in being one of the most effective methods to obtain results in a short time.

Even for the increase of muscle mass or other conditional properties such as strength, resistance or speed, specific workouts are necessary, programmed according to the objectives and the individual characteristics of each.

The diet alone, is not enough to achieve the objectives. A physical fitness program is also necessary in conjunction with nutritional considerations.

For example, if we are faced with a slender person who intends to increase their physical stature, we must not make the mistake, as I have often seen, to disproportionately increase the amount of calories in the diet.

In this way, fat alone will be what the increase in stature consists of, and the metabolic condition will be worsened in the process with be overexertion in the liver and kidney damage, as well as damage to organs, tissues and blood circulation, probably due to the uncontrolled and potentially inflammatory diet.

Note that body structure, or your somatotype, depends on several factors (structural and nervous), which are determined primarily by genetics and secondly by history, that emerges with the processes of growth and development. People who, for example, has never practiced a sport and at thirty years old decide to improve their own physical appearance, will hardly be able to obtain satisfactory results, because their physiology has been carved out over in time.[51,52]

In contrast, those who have had a sporting history of some kind, neglected perhaps for a few years, will likely fail to achieve satisfactory results in the resumption of training.

Having these basic concepts clearly understood, you can still obtain improvements, provided that physical activity is programmed with the right methodology: work in super series, giant series, forced reps, stripping, negative reps, etc. are all methods of work carried out to create hypertrophy and increased muscle mass.

The diet, in this case, should not disrupt the body, especially in a radical or sudden manner, but should cover the needs and increases of any requirements.

The increase in calories and/or the increase of protein, without the neuro-motor stimulation and training, can overload the organs and tissues, creating potential problems for the body. Overeating will result in an increase in body fat which is certainly not the intended objective.

If you want to get muscle growth you need to work well on the training principles, with the right recovery time, to give the muscles to opportunity to create the supercompensation (the benefits of the work done), increasing only moderately and only if the body actually requires it (increased sense of hunger) the amounts of food. [53, 54]

Our body if fed well communicates its needs. If the training has created the conditions for growth and muscle adaptation, the feeling of "hunger" will be felt, so you will have to slightly increase the amounts of food in order to meet energy needs.

This leads to an increase in the accompanying micro and macro nutrients necessary for growth and hypertrophy.

Not only is it the micronutrients that determine the "effects" in the body, but the overall micro elements and a well-balanced diet in general, as required in the Healthy Natural Diet.

HND PROGRAMS: INNOVATION FOR GUARANTEED RESULTS

Today, It is possible to obtain satisfactory results in just 10 days with an innovative and effective method: the HND program

These customized programs of varying duration are designed to improve lifestyle, focusing on nutrition, physical activity and meditation, key aspects in reaching the goal of being healthy. The HND routes are held in the island of Gran Canaria, an environment with an extraordinary climate, perfect to combine with a pleasant holiday.

They offer customized programs according to the needs and objectives by working daily with well-defined protocols. Activities include:

– Muscle toning and meditation

– Differentiated Daily Physical Activity:

  • Mobilization

  • Proprioception

  • Using equipment (rocker, kettlebell, trx, etc.).

  • Development of strength and power

  • Development of resistance

- Cooking course HND

- Shopping at the supermarket

- Lessons on nutrition

- Trekking around the island

The real added value is your chance to be followed daily by two professionals, to define the objectives, clarify doubts and be guided in the best way towards conscious change.

At the end of the trail you will have the information necessary to proceed in total autonomy but safeguarded by the professional support.

For more information, visit

www.healthynaturaldiet.eu

Bibliography

1. *Muggeo M, Bonora E. Diabetes and plurimetabolic syndrome. Pisa Pacini Editore, 2001*

2. *Shiraki K. Obesity as the core of the metabolic syndrome and the management of coronary heart disease. Curr Med Res Opin 2004; 20: 295-304*

3. *Ford ES, Giles WH, Dietz WH. Prevalence of metabolic syndrome among US adults. Finding from the third National Health and Nutrition Examination Survey. Jama 2002; 287: 356-9*

4. *Palaniappan L, Carnethon MR, Wang Y et al. Predictors of the incident metabolic syndrome in adults Diabetes care 2004: 27:788-93.*

5. *Lennerz B, Lennerz JK.Food Addiction, High-Glycemic-Index Carbohydrates, and Obesity. Clin Chem. 2018 Jan;64(1):64-71. doi: 10.1373/clinchem.2017.273532. Epub 2017 Nov 20.*

6. *Lemeshow AR1, Rimm EB2, Hasin DS3, Gearhardt AN4, Flint AJ5, Field AE6, Genkinger JM7.Food and beverage consumption and food addiction among women in the Nurses' Health Studies. Appetite. 2018 Feb 1;121:186-197. doi: 10.1016/j.appet.2017.10.038. Epub 2017 Nov 1.*

7. *DiNicolantonio JJ1, O'Keefe JH1, Wilson WL2.Sugar addiction: is it real? A narrative review. Br J Sports Med. 2017 Aug 23. pii: bjsports-2017-097971. doi: 10.1136/bjsports-2017-097971.*

8. *Baumgartner, R N, et al: bioelectric impedance for body composition. In Exercise and Sport Sciences Reviews. Vol.18. K.B. Pandolf and J.O. Hollozsy (Eds) Baltimore, Williams & Wilkens, 1990.*

9. *Borkan, G.A., et al: Profiles of selected hormones during menstrual cycles of teenages athletes. J.Appl.Physiol., 50:545, 1981.*

10. *Behnke, A.R., and Wilmore, J.H.: evaluation and regulation of Body Build and Composition, Englewood Cliffs, N.J., Prentice-Hall, 1974.*

11. *Bunt, J.C., et al: Impact of total body water fluctuations on estimation of body fat from body density. Med.Sci, Sport Exerc. 21:96, 1989.*

12. *Brooks.G.A: Physical activity and carbohydrate metabolism. In physical Activity Fitness and Health. C. Bouchard, et al. Eds, Champaign, IL, Human kinetics 1994.*

13. *Kiens, B, et al: Skeletal Muscle substrate utilization during submaximal exercise in man: Effect of Endurance training. J.Physiol., 469:459,1993.*

14. *Mudio, D.M., et al: Effects of dietary fat on metabolic adjustments to maximal VO2 and endurance in runners. Med. Sci. Sports Exerc. 26:81, 1994.*

15. *Fink J, Schoenfeld BJ, Nakazato K. The role of hormones in muscle hypertrophy. Phys Sportsmed. 2017 Nov 25:1-6.*

16. *SINU, Italian society of human nutrition. LARN, Levels of Nourishing and Nutrition Reference for the Italian population. IV Revision.*

17. *Paul Kouchakoff "The Influence of Food Cooking on the Blood Formula of Man of the Institute of Clinical Chemistry, Lausanne,*

Switzerland, Proceedings: First International Congress of Microbiology, Paris 1930.

18. *Elaine schrumpf, Helen charley texture of broccoli and carrots cooked by microwave energy first published: september 1975 full publication history doi: 10.1111/j.1365-2621.1975.*

19. Messina, Mangels, Messina.The Dietitian's Guide to Vegetarian Diets. Jones and Bartlett.

20. Welch AA[1], Shakya-Shrestha S, Lentjes MA, Wareham NJ, Khaw KT. Dietary intake and status of n-3 polyunsaturated fatty acids in a population of fish-eating and non-fish-eating meat-eaters, vegetarians, and vegans and the product-precursor ratio [corrected] of α-linolenic acid to long-chain n-3 polyunsaturated fatty acids: results from the EPIC-Norfolk cohort. Am J Clin Nutr. 2010 Nov;92(5):1040-51. doi: 10.3945/ajcn.2010.29457. Epub 2010 Sep 22.

21. DeFilippis, L Sperling, Understanding omega-3's, in Am Heart J, vol. 151, 2006, pp. 564-570.

22. Roncaglioni MC, Tombesi M, Avanzini F, et al., n-3 fatty acids in patients with multiple cardiovascular risk factors, in N. Engl. J. Med., vol. 368, n° 19, maggio 2013, pp. 1800–8, DOI:10.1056/NEJMoa1205409, PMID 23656645.

23. Cordeiro Sousa D[1], Ferreira Dos Santos G[2], Costa J[3], Vaz-Carneiro A[4].

24. Analysis of the Cochrane Review: Omega-3 Fatty Acids for the Treatment of Dementia. Cochrane Database Syst Rev. 2016;4:CD009002.Acta Med Port. 2017 Oct 31;30(10):671-674. doi: 10.20344/amp.9743. Epub 2017 Oct 31.

25. Agostoni C[1,2], Nobile M[3], Ciappolino V[4], Delvecchio G[5], Tesei A[6], Turolo S[7], Crippa A[8], Mazzocchi A[9], Altamura CA[10], Brambilla P[11,12].The Role of Omega-3 Fatty Acids in Developmental Psychopathology: A Systematic Review on Early Psychosis, Autism, and ADHD.Int J Mol Sci. 2017 Dec 4;18(12). pii: E2608. doi: 10.3390/ijms18122608.

26. Prokopiou E[1], Kolovos P[1], Kalogerou M[1], Neokleous A[1], Papagregoriou G[2], Deltas C[2], Malas S[3], Georgiou T[1].Therapeutic potential of omega-3 fatty acids supplementation in a mouse model of dry macular degeneration.BMJ Open Ophthalmol. 2017 Jun 19;1(1):e000056. doi: 10.1136/bmjophth-2016-000056. eCollection 2017.

27. www.scienzavegetariana.it

28. Sethi S[1], Ziouzenkova O, Ni H, Wagner DD, Plutzky J, Mayadas TN. Oxidized omega-3 fatty acids in fish oil inhibit leukocyte-endothelial interactions through activation of PPAR alpha. Blood. 2002 Aug 15;100(4):1340-6.

29. Fatati, Amerio, Dietetics e Nutrition, scientific thought Publisher: cap 6.114-116

30. GRAY LF, DANIEL LJ. Studies of Vitamin B12 in turnip greens.,J Nutr. 1959 Apr 10;67(4):623-34.

31. halsted ja, carroll j, rubert s.serum and tissue concentration of Vitamin b12 in certain pathologic states. n engl j med. 1959 mar 19;260(12):575-80

32. Mozafar J. Oertli Uptake of a microbially-produced Vitamin (B12) by soybean roots Plant and Soil January 1992, Volume 139, Issue 1, pp 23–30

33. Fumio Watanabe, Vitamin B12 Sources and Bioavailability, Experimental Biology and Medicine, N. 232(10), 2007, pp. 1266-1274

34. Stephen Walsh. Algae and B12 Filed 11 May 2012 in Internet Archive. Published online: 7 June 2002.
(IT) Translation edited by Luciana Baroni.

35. M A Juillerat M B Reddy S R Lynch S A Dassenko J D Cook Soy protein, phytate, and iron absorption in humans The American Journal of Clinical Nutrition, Volume 56, Issue 3, 1 September 1992, Pages 573–578, https://doi.org/10.1093/ajcn/56.3.573

36. L Hallberg L Rossander A B Skånberg Phytates and the inhibitory effect of bran on iron absorption in man The American Journal of Clinical Nutrition, Volume 45, Issue 5, 1 May 1987, Pages 988–996,https://doi.org/10.1093/ajcn/45.5.988

37. Chaudhari AS[1], Raghuvanshi R[1], Kumar GN[2]. Genetically engineered Escherichia coli Nissle 1917 synbiotic counters fructose-induced metabolic syndrome and iron deficiency. Appl Microbiol Biotechnol. 2017 Jun;101(11):4713-4723. doi: 10.1007/s00253-017-8207-7. Epub 2017 Mar 10.

38. Morck TA, Lynch SR, Cook JD. Inhibition of food iron absorption by coffee. Am J Clin Nutr. 1983 Mar;37(3):416-20.

39. Hallberg L[1], Hulthén L. Prediction of dietary iron absorption: an algorithm for calculating absorption and bioavailability of dietary iron. Am J Clin Nutr. 2000 May;71(5):1147-60.

40. Yi-ChiaHuangPh.D.Woei-JyueLinMSChien-HsiangChengM.D.Kuo-HsiungSuPh.D. Nutrient intakes and iron status of healthy young vegetarians and nonvegetarians Institute of Nutritional Science and School of Nutrition, Chung Shan Medical and Dental College, and Veterans General Hospital, Taichung, Taiwan, ROC Accepted 2 October 1998, Available online 29 July 1999.

41. Osis D, Coffey J, Spencer H. Mineral and trace element content of vegetarian diets. J Am Coll Nutr. 1984;3(1):3-11.

42. Zeng SB1, Weng H, Zhou M, Duan XL, Shen XF, Zeng XT. Long-Term Coffee Consumption and Risk of Gastric Cancer: A PRISMA-Compliant Dose-Response Meta-Analysis of Prospective Cohort Studies. Medicine (Baltimore). 2015 Sep;94(38)

43. Morales-Suárez-Varela M1,2, Nohr EA3, Olsen J4, Bech BH5.Potential combined effects of maternal smoking and coffee intake on foetal death within the Danish National Birth Cohort. Eur J Public Health. 2017 Dec 22.

44. Gonzalez de Mejia E1, Ramirez-Mares MV2. Impact of caffeine and coffee on our health. Trends Endocrinol Metab. 2014 Oct;25(10):489-92.

45. Godos J1, Pluchinotta FR, Marventano S, Buscemi S, Li Volti G, Galvano F, Grosso G.Coffee components and cardiovascular risk: beneficial and detrimental effects. Int J Food Sci Nutr. 2014 Dec;65(8):925-36.

46. *Rodríguez-Artalejo F1,2,3, López-García E1,2,3.Coffee Consumption and Cardiovascular Disease: A Condensed Review of Epidemiological Evidence and Mechanisms.J Agric Food Chem. 2018 Jan 10.*

47. *Kashino I[1], Akter S[1], Mizoue T[1], Sawada N[2], Kotemori A[2], Matsuo K[3,4], Oze I[3], Ito H[3,4], Naito M[5], Nakayama T[6], Kitamura Y[7], Tamakoshi A[8], Tsuji I[9], Sugawara Y[9], Inoue M[2], Nagata C[10], Sadakane A[11], Tanaka K[12], Tsugane S[2], Shimazu T[2]; Research Group for the Development and Evaluation of Cancer Prevention Strategies in Japan. Coffee drinking and colorectal cancer and its subsites: A pooled analysis of 8 cohort studies in Japan.Int J Cancer. 2018 Feb 15.*

48. *Assessment of moderate coffee consumption and risk of epithelial ovarian cancer: a Mendelian randomization study. Int J Epidemiol. 2017 Nov 25. doi: 10.1093/ije/dyx236.*

49. *Narita S[1], Saito E[2,3], Sawada N[3], Shimazu T[3], Yamaji T[3], Iwasaki M[3], Sasazuki S[3], Noda M[4,5], Inoue M[2,3], Tsugane S[3].Coffee Consumption and Lung Cancer Risk: The Japan Public Health Center-Based Prospective Study.J Epidemiol. 2017 Nov 18. doi: 10.2188/jea.JE20160191*

50. *Watson EJ1, Banks S1, Coates AM2, Kohler MJ1. The Relationship Between Caffeine, Sleep, and Behavior in Children. J Clin Sleep Med. 2017 Apr 15;13(4):533-543.*

51. *Watson EJ1, Coates AM2, Kohler M3, Banks S4. Caffeine Consumption and Sleep Quality in Australian Adults. Nutrients. 2016 Aug 4;8(8)*

52. *Dangayach NS, O'Phelan KH.Understanding the Functional Neuroanatomical basis of Meditation for Improving Patient Wellness*

and Outcomes. World Neurosurg. 2018 Feb 16. pii: S1878-8750(18)30334-6. doi: 10.1016/j.wneu.2018.02.063.]

53. *Lopez G[1], Chaoul A[1], Powers-James C[1], Spelman A[1], Wei Q[1], Engle R[1], Hashmi Y[1], Bruera E[1], Cohen L[2]. A pragmatic evaluation of symptom distress after group meditation for cancer patients and caregivers: a preliminary report. J Pain Symptom Manage. 2018 Feb 5. pii: S0885-3924(18)30038-1. doi: 10.1016/j.jpainsymman.2018.01.018.*

54. *Ho RTH[1,2], Wan AHY[3,4], Chan JSM[4], Ng SM[4], Chung KF[5], Chan CLW[4]. Study protocol on comparative effectiveness of mindfulness meditation and qigong on psychophysiological outcomes for patients with colorectal cancer: a randomized controlled trial. BMC Complement Altern Med. 2017; 17: 390. Published online 2017 Aug 8. doi: 10.1186/s12906-017-1898-6*

55. *Chang YY[1,2], Wang LY[3], Liu CY[1,3], Chien TJ[1,3], Chen IJ[1,3], Hsu CH[1,3,4]. The Effects of a Mindfulness Meditation Program on Quality of Life in Cancer Outpatients. Integr Cancer Ther. 2017 Feb 1:1534735417693359. doi: 10.1177/1534735417693359.*

56. *OMS-WHO. Global health risk: mortality and burden of disease attributable to selected major risk. Geneva: WHO, 2009.*

57. *OMS-WHO. Global recommendation on physical activity for health. Geneva: WHO, 2010.*

58. *Spada R, Giampietro M. Physical activity as a therapy tool. In: Gentile MG, ed. Updates in clinical nutrition. Volume 14. Rome: the Thinking Scientific Publisher, 2006.*

59. *D. Barbieri. Basic elements for functional training, the game of iron. Pu. Calzetti Mariucci 2013.*

60. D. Barbieri. *Athletic preparation. Strength, speed and power for the sport,* Ed. Elika, Cesena (FC) 2008.

61. Williams PT- Hight density lipoprotein cholesterol and other risk factors for coronary heart disease in female runners. N Engl J Med 1996; 334:1298-303.

62. Smith JK, Dykes R Douglas JE, Krishnaswamy G, Berk S. Long term exercise and atherogenic activity of blood mononuclear cells in persona t risk of developing ischemic heart disease. JAMA 1999; 281:1722-7.

63. P Vitulli G.D. et al. Physical activity and aging. Exercise training and aging. G.Gerontol 2012-60:172-181.

64. Hanson PG, Flaherty DK. Immunological responses to training in conditioned runners. Clin Sci (Lond). 1981 Feb;60(2):225-8.

65. Viti A, Muscettola M, Paulesu L, Bocci V, Almi A. Effect of exercise on plasma interferon levels. J Appl Physiol (1985). 1985 Aug;59(2):426-8.

66. Chad KE, Wenger HA. The effect of exercise duration on the exercise and post-exercise oxygen consumption. Canadian Journal of Sport Science, 1988. 13(4), 204-207.

67. Krzentowski et al. Metabolic adaptations in post-exercise recovery. Clin Physiol. 1982 Aug;2(4):277-88.

68. Folch et al. Metabolic response to small and large 13C-labelled pasta meals following rest or exercise in man. Br J Nutr. 2001 Jun;85(6):671-80.

69. Giampietro M. Nutrition for exercise and sport. Rome: scientific thought Publisher, 2005.

70. Schoenfeld B. MS, CSCS. Does Cardio After an Overnight Fast Maximize Fat Loss?. Strength & Conditioning Journal. Feb 2011 - Volume 33 - Issue 1 - pp 23-25

71. Helms et al. Recommendations for natural bodybuilding contest preparation: resistance and cardiovascular training. J Sports Med Phys Fitness. 2014 Jul 7.

72. Coyle EF. Substrate utilization during exercise in active people. Am J Clin Nutr. 1995 Apr;61(4 Suppl):968S-979S.

73. Venkatraman JT, Pendergast DR. Effect of dietary intake on immune function in athletes. Sports Med. 2002;32(5):323-37.

74. Marcello Lostia. Models of the mind, models of the person. The two souls of psychology. Taylor & Francis, 1994. p. 124. ISBN 8809205561.

75. Vincenzo Mezzogiorno Human morphotypology. PICCIN, 1981. p. 244. ISBN 8821209180

76. T. Jeff Chandler, Lee E. Brown. Conditioning for Strength and Human Performance. Lippincott Williams & Wilkins, 2008. pp. 284. ISBN 0781745942.

77. Fleck SJ, Kraemer WJ. Designing Resistance Training Programs. Human Kinetics 1, 2004. ISBN 0736042571.

Social Media

To stay up to date

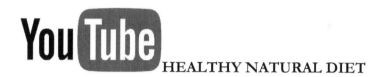 HEALTHY NATURAL DIET

HEALTHYNATURALDIETOFFICIAL

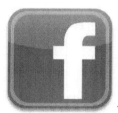

HEALTHY NATURAL DIET

34908641R00103

Printed in Poland
by Amazon Fulfillment
Poland Sp. z o.o., Wrocław